TESTOSTERONE
MATTERS . . . MORE!

THE SECRET TO
HEALTHY AGING
IN WOMEN

GARY DONOVITZ, MD

Published by Wheatmark®
2030 East Speedway Boulevard, Suite 106
Tucson, Arizona 85719 USA
www.wheatmark.com

ISBN: 978-1-62787-800-5 (paperback)
ISBN: 978-1-62787-801-2 (ebook)
LCCN: 2020907338

Bulk ordering discounts are available through Wheatmark, Inc.
For more information, email orders@wheatmark.com or call 1-888-934-0888.

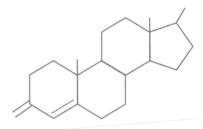

CONTENTS

ACKNOWLEDGMENTS

To my wife, Lani, she has inspired me to keep changing healthcare and fight the fight for women's health. She is my best friend with whom I found happiness within myself and our relationship. She is an incredible life partner with whom I enjoyed sharing the journey of the creation of *Testosterone Matters...More!* and what is yet to be in the next chapter of our life.

To my daughter, Mandy, who has been such a great protégé in my quest to change healthcare. She has a heart of gold and is the most caring nurse practitioner I know. Her contributions to our veterans in heading up the PTSD study changed hundreds of lives. The Institute for Hormonal Balance has never been in more capable hands. She has built an amazing research center for BioTE to train our practitioners. Mandy has been my cheerleader, literally, for years and is the bright light in my soul forever.

To my son Chase, although he is 12 years old, he has told me how proud he is that his dad has been able to help so many people feel better. Changing healthcare, writing, and research have taken valuable time away from him, and his heartfelt understanding means so much. He understands BioTE and still asks questions that I have not been able to answer yet!

Thank you to Ann Wixon who helped me tell my stories and made them coherent for all to understand. Ann has such an ability to transfer medical content into words and phrases that deliver the message for both practitioners and patients to understand.

Nancy Mamann, thank you for help in coordinating the cover shoot and really giving that special look to *Testosterone Matters... More!*

Sam Henrie and Wheatmark Publishing, thank you for making the trip from manuscript to finished product a seamless, easy journey.

There are others who are part of the journey and helped me see things through the eyes of women. So many people right now have, through gender bias, tried to take away testosterone for use in women. For the hundreds of thousands of women who will read this book, I applaud you for your efforts in the future to make sure no one takes away your most important hormone.

Finally, to my all patients who have trusted me to help them for the past thirty-five years, thank you for all your referrals!

FOREWORD

Are women's health and hormone replacement therapy (HRT) under attack?

Dr. Donovitz has been on my podcast many times. Women's health and especially HRT are topics I continue to address because they are too often marginalized. I have clinically seen the suffering needlessly endured when these issues are left unaddressed. I am equally well aware of the controversies swirling about this subject.

In the 1990s, estrogen therapy (ET) became the standard of treatment of the almost six hundred thousand women a year in the United States undergoing hysterectomy, and more than 90 percent of hysterectomized women in their fifties used ET. I had patients in their eighties and nineties who had been on hormone replacement since forever, and I noticed their cognition seemed to be superior and their risk of vascular events seemed to be less. However, in July 2002, the Women's Health Initiative (WHI) published the results of the Estrogen Plus Progestin Trial, announcing that it had been terminated ahead of schedule because of adverse effects in the women receiving hormones versus those who received placebo. That's when the tailspin for women's health began. Many of my colleagues were skeptical of these results. We had patients and saw firsthand how beneficial HRT could be. But what we were all told was, "If you believe that, it's because you are seeing too small a sample, and we have this huge sample, and you have to go with the science as it is." We were warned that not doing so made us purely witchdoctors.

As physicians, "Do no harm" is drilled into our heads. It's funny: I remember when the WHI report came out, that phrase, "Do no harm," was ringing loudly in my head because bringing women off these hormones was going to do harm in spite of the WHI "science." At the time, I relied on collaboration with my patients. I said, "Look, here's the science as we understand it, and I'm being told I have to follow the science and the evidence, which I always do, but something isn't right. What would you like to do?" Many women said, "No way! Don't even think about changing anything."

Those were the lucky women. In 2013, the *American Journal of Public Health* published a study called "The Mortality Toll of Estrogen Avoidance: An Analysis of Excess Deaths among Hysterectomized Women Aged 50 to 59 Years." The results: "Over a 10-year span, starting in 2002, a minimum of 18,601 and as many as 91,610 postmenopausal women died prematurely because of avoidance of estrogen therapy." It was only one study, to be sure, but an attention grabber.

You can't allow the sea of misinformation to have influence and control over your health. There's a shroud of secrecy and shame around menopause—and, frankly, the research dollars that have been spent on testosterone and women focus mainly on libido. You might argue that limiting the clinical response to libido is subtly (or not so subtly) misogynistic. In fact, the only thing testosterone has been approved for is hypoactive sexual desire disorder.

Testosterone does improve sexual health, and when sexual health is good, libido, desire, and mood improve. While that's happening, there is some evidence that testosterone is also protecting your heart, your brain, your bones, your mood, and your muscles and joints. There's also a vital connection to thyroid health. It is difficult to understand why estrogen often seems to be the only option and the hormone of choice to replace hormones in post-menopausal women when testosterone also treats more symptoms of menopause that estrogen (estradiol) may not control.

Like Dr. Donovitz, I'm a champion for women's health. That's where the real value of this book lies. So many other books are merely a compilation of patient anecdotes. Dr. Donovitz provides scientific evidence that is based on clinical studies and on which you can make a decision about the course of your own health. Why not feel your best no matter what your age?

—Drew Pinsky, MD (known nationally as "Dr. Drew")

IF ESTROGEN MATTERS, WHY DOES TESTOSTERONE MATTER MORE?

If you Google "testosterone," you will get over 49,300,000 results—almost all for men. Even *Merriam-Webster* defines testosterone as a hormone made by the testes that is responsible for inducing and maintaining male secondary sex characteristics.

So if testosterone is all about being a strong, healthy, and manly man, as a woman, do you need it or even want it?

Great question! This book will surprise you, enlighten you, and be life-changing for you, your family, and your female friends.

But if your doctor or medical professional has never mentioned testosterone (and my guess is that they have not), how do you even know if you need more of it? Here's the health assessment I ask every patient to fill out:

Which of the following symptoms currently apply to you (in the last two weeks)? Please mark the appropriate box for each symptom. For symptoms that do not currently apply or no longer apply, mark "none."

Symptom	None	Mild	Moderate	Severe	Very Severe
Score =	0	1	2	3	4
1 Hot flashes					
2 Sweating (night sweats or increased episodes of sweating)					
3 Sleep problems (difficulty falling asleep or sleeping through the night, or waking up too early)					
4 Depressive mood (feeling down, sad, or on the verge of tears, or lacking drive)					
5 Irritability (mood swings, aggression, easily angered)					
6 Anxiety (inner restlessness, feeling panicky, feeling nervous, inner tension)					
7 Physical exhaustion (general decrease in muscle strength or endurance, decrease in work performance, fatigue, or lack of energy, stamina, or motivation)					
8 Sexual problems (change in sexual desire, in sexual activity and/or orgasm and satisfaction)					
9 Bladder problems (difficulty in urinating, increased need to urinate, incontinence)					
10 Vaginal symptoms (sensation of dryness or burning in vagina, difficulty with sexual intercourse)					
11 Joint and muscular symptoms (joint pain or swelling, muscle weakness, poor recovery after exercise)					
12 Difficulties with memory					
13 Problems with thinking, concentrating, or reasoning					
14 Difficulty learning new things					
15 Trouble thinking of the right word to describe persons, places, or things when speaking					
16 Increase in frequency or intensity of headaches or migraines					
17 Hair loss, thinning or change in texture of hair					
18 Feel cold all the time or have cold hands or feet					
19 Weight gain or difficulty losing weight despite diet and exercise					
20 Dry or wrinkled skin					

Table 1. Modified Female Health Assessment

If your total score is 14 or more and you were sitting in my office, I would advise you that you most likely are a candidate for hormone optimization therapy. I would also suggest we evaluate your hormone levels with a simple blood test.

Most patients I have discussed hormone replacement with over the past thirty-five years assume I am talking about optimizing their levels of estrogen, but that could not be further from the truth and not always what you actually need to feel better.

Here's the thing: most physicians and medical societies have focused for years on the necessity of estrogen for symptoms of menopause. In February 2018, Dr. Blumel and colleagues found that if you scored above 14 on a similar questionnaire, you most likely required hormone replacement for symptoms of menopause. What was striking in their study was that hot flashes and vaginal dryness were not the most common symptoms of that season of your life. What was even more interesting in Dr. Rebecca Glazer's study on the validated Menopause Rating Scale questionnaire (a very similar instrument to the health assessment in Table 1 to measure the severity of symptoms of pre- and postmenopausal women) was that all of these symptoms responded to testosterone therapy.

You see, the score you receive from this questionnaire is more often than not an SOS from your endocrine system—your hormones—saying that your testosterone is too low. What this means to you is that in addition to suffering from hot flashes, night sweats, weight gain, joint pain, decreased sex drive, insomnia, mood swings, and anxiety, you may be at an increased risk for Alzheimer's disease, heart disease, breast cancer, and osteoporosis.

Now I'm not trying to scare you, but the medical community has seen these studies and many more—yet remains silent. The American College of Obstetrics and Gynecology has failed to incorporate testosterone therapy into its advanced courses in HRT.

The Endocrine Society took a position that testosterone for women was untested and not proven safe and effective. This position failed to examine the literature published around the world for the past nearly eighty years. I went to the Food and Drug Administration to get our hormone pellets approved for women. The committee told me they were not interested in its use for women . . . period! Since there are absolutely zero medical reasons to support that decision, you've kind of got to ask: What are they really afraid of—women taking control of their bodies, protecting their health, and feeling a bit friskier? It does make you wonder.

The bottom line is that testosterone is safe and effective, and the benefits are extraordinary.

As you read this book, I hope the experiences that patients and practitioners were kind enough to share will resonate and you find yourself in one of the chapters. Feeling your best, no matter your age, is important for you, your family, and your job. This book will hopefully be a pathway out of the fog of menopause and may offer a clear solution to overcome many of the chronic ailments you have suffered from. As you know from my first book, *Age Healthier . . . Live Happier*, now with over three hundred thousand copies in print, I want you to feel your best and not be on multiple pills to treat all of these symptoms you are experiencing. Pills may not get to the root cause of the problem and may cause severe side effects that degrade the quality of your life. You may not need them in your medicine cabinet when you get your hormones optimized, especially when you optimize your testosterone.

One hundred years ago, the end of being fertile and reproducing was the end of a woman's life. In 1930, only half of women lived longer than fifty years old. In 2020, you can expect to live forty-plus years beyond the onset of menopause. And without proper hormone optimization individualized for you, you can expect to be miserable during most of it!

If this sounds like there is hope for you to live happier while you age healthier, keep reading. It is not that your doctor told you the wrong story all these years. It is not that your family misled you on the risk of HRT. It is not that the media meant to scare you about hormone therapy. Unfortunately, in each case, you only heard part of the story.

I share the whole story with you so you can make a fair and independent decision about managing *all* of your hormones during perimenopause and menopause.

You are you again.

Let's begin our journey into *Testosterone Matters . . . More!* by looking at the top 10 myths about testosterone and women.

1. Testosterone is a male hormone.

Nothing could be further from the truth.

Throughout your life, testosterone is your most abundant active hormone. Women make more testosterone daily than they do estrogen; in fact, in your twenties and thirties, you made fifty times more testosterone than estrogen.

This is because testosterone plays a role in protecting every organ and system in your body. Indeed, there are receptors to receive your testosterone throughout your body (see Figure 1). It is through this complex binding of your testosterone hormone to all these areas throughout your body that your overall well-being and quality of life are maintained.

In August 2018, the "International Consensus Paper of Testosterone Use in Women" was published in *Medicina y Salud Publica*. One of the resolutions in this landmark paper was that testosterone is the most important hormone for women no matter what decade of life they are visiting. Stated more simply, as you progress through the seasons of your life, testosterone is your source of youth and vitality. More importantly, even though most women focus on estrogen or the lack thereof, it turns out that testosterone matters more than estrogen.

Figure 1. Androgen Receptors in Females

Androgen Receptors
Hair follicle, skin, scalp
Brain, spinal cord, nerves, eyes, ears
Thyroid, endocrine glands
Cardiovascular
* Breast *
Pulmonary (Lungs, bronchi)
GI tract, liver, pancreas kidneys, adrenals
Uterus, vagina, bladder
Sexual organs
Muscle (smooth/striated)
Bone, bone marrow, joints
Fat

2. Testosterone's only role in women is sex drive and libido.

Although many physicians and medical societies continue to state that the only benefit of testosterone is for peri- and postmenopausal women with low libido, and the only FDA indication for its use in women is hypoactive sexual dysphoric disorder, they are missing the more important benefits.

Remember from the androgen receptors in females (Figure 1) that there are testosterone receptors in almost all tissues. Most women begin losing testosterone in their mid-twenties.

In fact, the International Consensus group of experts in bioidentical HRT agreed that testosterone deficiency is a clinical syndrome. (A clinical syndrome represents a typical constellation of physical and laboratory findings that may be seen as part of a primary disease process.) As such, as you lose testosterone, you may experience lack of well-being; fatigue; insomnia; weight gain; joint pain; brain fog; mood changes like irritability, anxiety, and depression; urinary incontinence; and night sweats.

You can see that the loss of testosterone (a.k.a. androgen deficiency) is a health condition that makes itself known with a variety of symptoms; in fact, this is truer than for any other hormone.

The medical community needs to recognize androgen deficiency, screen women for it yearly starting in their mid-twenties, and help women feel their best at every age and stage of life without overmedicating them for all the symptoms the lack of testosterone causes.

3. Testosterone masculinizes women.

This myth always puzzles me even though I hear it shared as a concern all the time. It's been recognized for over sixty-five years that true masculinization in women is not possible unless long-term and supraphysiologic levels of testosterone are achieved; however, this is not considered HRT.

When you were at your peak in terms of testosterone production—your mid- to late twenties—you certainly were *not* masculine. That's because the amount of testosterone in your system was appropriate for you as a woman. You felt good, energetic, and on top of your game.

As your testosterone levels are dropping, what's happening? You don't feel good. You don't feel like you anymore.

Testosterone, at the right level for you, may restore you! It's not going to make you suddenly enjoy football, chug beer, and smash the beer can on your forehead.

Here's the thing: in low doses, testosterone does not increase facial hair growth or cause clitoral enlargement. Mild engorgement of the clitoris is possible as testosterone dilates the blood vessels in the clitoris. However, masculinization is not possible in the usual doses of bioidentical testosterone required to optimize your hormones.

The delivery method is key, and the most stable physiologic doses occur with subcutaneous pellet therapy, while using testosterone cream often results in much higher blood levels, leading to more unwanted side effects.

Synthetic androgens like the drug danazol have resulted in cases of clitoromegaly (unusual enlargement of the clitoris), another reason I don't recommend synthetic testosterone to my patients.

Furthermore, animal studies have failed to show any adverse effects on female fetuses. In pregnancy, a woman makes up to four times as much testosterone as when she is not pregnant. The placenta protects the fetus from these higher levels. You can be assured that optimal therapy with bioidentical testosterone has no masculinizing effect on you or your fetus.

4. Testosterone causes hoarseness and voice changes.

A lot of women say, "Oh, well, I don't want to take testosterone. I don't want my voice to deepen. I don't want to sound like my husband."

But the reality is hoarseness and voice changes occur as a natural part of aging. In fact, more than 30 percent of women will deepen their voice or develop hoarseness sometime in their life. This may be from seasonal allergies, overusing your voice (e.g., yelling at your husband or children), inflammation of the vocal cords, smoking, or polyps. Studies in the literature have shown no evidence that testosterone causes these voice changes. The results of a twelve-month study published in 2016 state, "Despite 'reports' in the literature, and urban legends on the Internet, there is a lack of quality evidence supporting that testosterone-replacement therapy negatively affects the female voice."

Often, women with low testosterone have hoarseness because they have lost the anti-inflammatory protection seen with normal levels of testosterone. If your voice is an asset to your profession, there is no evidence that testosterone will jeopardize this.

5. Testosterone causes hair loss.

Rest assured that optimizing your testosterone will not make you lose your hair, and less than 1 percent of the women for whom I have optimized their testosterone have hair thinning.

Approximately one-third of women will lose hair as they age. I have personally seen hair regrow in these women. That's because testosterone stimulates hair follicles. A study published in 2012 evaluated the effect of subcutaneous testosterone therapy on scalp hair growth in 285 female patients. Seventy-six percent had hair thinning prior to treatment, and 48 percent of those women *reported hair regrowth* while on testosterone therapy.

There is a more active testosterone hormone called dihydrotestosterone, and it is this hormone that contributes to male pattern hair loss. If you are obese or have prediabetes or diabetes, you can make more of this hormone and perhaps develop hair thinning. But the most common cause for hair loss in women is low thyroid hormone levels.

6. Testosterone has adverse effects on the heart.

I was taught in medical school that estrogen protected the heart in women and that's why women outlived their male counterparts. If this were completely the case, why does one in seven women die from heart disease during pre-menopause? The answer: it is because they have been losing testosterone—in many cases, since age twenty-five—and twenty or more years later, their testosterone levels are too low to offer proper cardiovascular protection and combat the silent killer: inflammation.

There is overwhelming evidence that testosterone protects your heart. Women who have low testosterone have more plaque in their blood vessels and a decreased exercise performance. In addition, testosterone has a beneficial effect on your lipids, both cholesterol and triglycerides. The bottom line for you: cardiovascular disease is the number-one killer of women, and testosterone is heart protective.

7. Testosterone causes liver damage.

Once again, a myth with no support in clinical studies. If you use bioidentical testosterone to combat testosterone deficiency as you age, there are no adverse effects on your liver. In addition, subcutaneous pellets are metabolized through your kidneys, not your liver. Pellets also bypass your stomach, so you absorb more of what you're given.

Even more good news is that non-oral testosterone—subcutaneous pellets or cream—does not increase your risk of blood clots. So using subcutaneous pellets or creams is acceptable even if you have had a history of a blood clot after pregnancy or fracture or other reasons.

8. Testosterone causes aggression.

Testosterone therapy actually decreases irritability, anxiety, and depression. Studies in medical literature have shown up to a 90 percent reduction in irritability, aggressive behavior, and anxiety in patients who had testosterone replacement therapy because they suffered from low testosterone. Imagine how the quality of your life could be improved once you are not having to take anxiety medications and antidepressants.

9. Testosterone may increase the risk of breast cancer.

My experience over the past thirty-five years has consistently been that women in general fear HRT because they are afraid of getting breast cancer from the hormones their bodies are craving. In his book *Estrogen Matters*, Avrum Bluming, MD, an oncologist and an investigator at the National Institutes of Health, clearly debunks the myth that estrogen causes breast cancer. He also shows that taking estrogen can improve the quality of women's lives.

In this book, we show you that testosterone does not increase the risk of breast cancer. Moreover, testosterone is breast protective. It not only helps prevent breast cancer but has also been shown to be therapeutic in patients who already have breast cancer. Allaying a woman's fear of breast cancer means that so many of you reading this book who thought you had to suffer from the symptoms of pre- and post-menopause can now enjoy life again . . . no need to fear the T!

10. The safety of testosterone use in women has not been established.

With all the benefits of testosterone therapy, I know you still have concerns about long-term safety. Get ready to breathe a sigh of relief. The safety of non-oral testosterone has been well established.

You probably didn't know that, for the past eighty years, testosterone has been used around the world to safely treat the symptoms of menopause. The fact that 95 percent of patients stay on testosterone therapy delivered by subcutaneous pellet implants is a testament to its efficacy and safety. No other HRT, not even estrogen, has this long a track record, life-changing benefits, and minimal side effects. Again, that's why testosterone matters . . . more!

How much better do you feel knowing that the uninformed and the press have propagated these myths limiting your future health? Now you know that you can safely get your life back, age healthier, and feel amazing again. Your world no longer has to be one of foggy gray typified by testosterone deficiency. Your world can be one of brilliant hues and jewel tones with your testosterone optimized.

Enjoy each of the following chapters. Find yourself, your family members, and your friends, and then get them reading *Testosterone Matters . . . More!* Enjoy the journey; the seasons of your life just got brighter.

2

TESTOSTERONE AND MENOPAUSE

Can you help me feel better?

Patient Testimonial

It's crippling to my life, my relationship, and my work. I was forty-two and had a hysterectomy for fibroid tumors. Over the next few months, my life went into a tailspin. I was gaining weight, my sex drive was nonexistent, my anxiety was escalating, and I was depressed. In addition, I was having hot flashes and vaginal dryness. I just felt broken. Paralyzed. I don't know where my energetic, happy person went. My husband thought he had lost his fun-loving wife. My doctor tried to treat me with synthetic estrogen pills. If anything, this made me feel worse. I went elsewhere and was placed on antidepressants. I felt like a zombie. They added diet pills for my weight gain, which stopped me from eating, and my metabolism slowed. How could I exercise with no food intake? My OB/GYN tried me on more hormone pills and then patches. I truly felt no better. My marriage was on the rocks, and to top it off, my husband got transferred for his job. New city, new house, no friends, and symptoms worsening. By the grace of God, I met a doctor who knew the answer. I needed my testosterone optimized. OMG, that was it! Off the diet pills, off the antide-

pressants, and my life was back. My husband and I got our
marriage back. I will never be without my testosterone again.

I went out to California in 2018 to give a talk to an OB/GYN Group. They were supposed to have food there. All they had was a Costco cheese tray. Really, that's not food. I was supposed to have dinner. After six hours of teaching, I went to the bar and got some bar food and a glass of wine.

A lady walked up and said, "Hey, what do you do?"

I said, "I'm a doctor."

"What kind of doctor?"

"OB/GYN."

She said, "Oh, listen, I have horrible hot flashes, terrible hot flashes. Fifteen a day. I can't work. I'm disabled. By the way, I'm here at this party outside, and I carry a fan in my bag."

I was thinking, *Oh my god. What's happening here?*

"Oh, it's starting now," she said and started sweating everywhere, all over my coat and everything. She was fanning herself.

I said, "What are you doing?"

She answered, "This is my life."

"Well, why don't you get some hormones?"

"Because they cause cancer."

"Really? What if that is not true?" I asked.

"Well, then, why hasn't anybody told me that?"

"I don't know."

"Can you help me?" she asked.

I said, "Yes, I can."

Here's the thing: menopause matters. This woman is fifty-seven years old. She looks older because she hasn't been on hormones. She's staring down at thirty more years potentially in menopause, and if she hadn't bumped into me at a bar, she may well have lived all thirty of them in total misery.

Why?

Because in 1991, the National Heart, Lung, and Blood Institute, part of the National Institute of Health (NIH), launched the Women's Health Initiative (WHI), focusing on women's health. More than 160,000 post-menopausal women ages fifty to seventy-nine participated in the fifteen-year study. Know what they discovered? Women whose doctors had put them on synthetic estrogen and synthetic progestin, in the form of a pill they took orally, had terrible side effects including an increased risk of breast cancer, heart disease, stroke, blood clots, and urinary incontinence.

Everyone froze. It's almost as if their brains disconnected. What did the medical community do to help these women? Practitioners told them, "You don't need hormones."

Eighty percent of women stopped taking their hormones. Practitioners quit giving them hormones. And because of that, we lost a whole generation of women. Tens of thousands of women died because they didn't take their estrogen. Yet those doctors who did the study are still restating their data and admitting their mistakes but have been unable to reverse the fears regarding the use of HRT and the mysterious risks they sensationalized.

Even more women were virtually disabled by menopause, aging them faster and robbing them of energy and vitality. As this woman in the bar said, "I've lost ten years of my life." Through fear and hesitancy to prescribe HRT and the lack of training in hormone optimization, women suffered an increased risk of Alzheimer's disease, heart disease, osteoporosis, diabetes, and probably breast cancer.

You do need hormones. You most definitely need testosterone. How many more years of your life are you willing to lose?

If you answered, "Not one more," keep reading—because if you're peri- or postmenopausal, testosterone is going to change your life.

Why your testosterone levels are too low.

Testosterone production in women comes from three sources: your ovaries, your adrenal glands, and then conversion from other circulating androgens in the bloodstream. Testosterone starts decreasing very early on, and, by the fifth decade, by age forty, a woman has lost half of her testosterone production. Androgen production from the adrenal glands declines, and testosterone production from the ovary remains relatively intact after menopause. Adrenal secretion of androstenedione declines by 50 percent, resulting in a significant reduction in peripheral conversion of testosterone at menopause. Additionally, women who have undergone bilateral oophorectomy experience a 50 percent further reduction in testosterone levels.

As if that weren't enough, we now know that exposure to endocrine-disrupting chemicals (EDCs) also reduces testosterone. A study published in the Endocrine Society's *Journal of Clinical Endocrinology & Metabolism (JCEM)* examined phthalate (a chemical to make plastics soft) exposure and testosterone levels in 2,208 people who participated and found that in women ages forty to sixty, increased phthalate concentrations were associated with a 10.8 to 24 percent decline in testosterone levels.

Another study, reported online in the journal *PLOS One*, revealed that women whose bodies have high levels of EDCs experience menopause two to four years earlier than those with lower levels of these chemicals.

Where are these EDCs hiding? They're found in plastics, common household items, pharmaceuticals, and personal-care products including lotions, perfumes, makeup, nail polish, liquid soap, and hairspray.

I thought my symptoms were because of low estrogen. You mean I need testosterone?

You're not alone. Most women believe it's the estrogen replacement that matters; however, as you will see, testosterone matters . . . more!

There is a great questionnaire called the Menopause Rating Scale (MRS), which was developed by Rebecca Glaser, MD, to determine if testosterone administered by subcutaneous pellets alone was effective for the relief of hormone deficiency symptoms in both pre- and postmenopausal women. Three hundred pre- and postmenopausal women were asked to complete the questionnaire before any treatment (to establish a baseline) and again three months after their first insertion of the subcutaneous testosterone pellet.

R. Glaser et al. / Maturitas 68 (2011) 355–361

Symptoms:	none	mild	moderate	severe	extremely severe
Score =	0	1	2	3	4
1. Hot flashes, sweating (episodes of sweating)	☐	☐	☐	☐	☐
2. Heart discomfort (unusual awareness of heart beat, heart skipping, heart racing, tightness)	☐	☐	☐	☐	☐
3. Sleep problems (difficulty in falling asleep, difficulty in sleeping through the night, waking up early)	☐	☐	☐	☐	☐
4. Depressive mood (feeling down, sad, on the verge of tears, lack of drive, mood swings)	☐	☐	☐	☐	☐
5. Irritability (feeling nervous, inner tension, feeling aggressive)	☐	☐	☐	☐	☐
6. Anxiety (inner restlessness, feeling panicky)	☐	☐	☐	☐	☐
7. Physical and mental exhaustion (general decrease in performance, impaired memory, decrease in concentration, forgetfulness)	☐	☐	☐	☐	☐
8. Sexual problems (change in sexual desire, in sexual activity and satisfaction)	☐	☐	☐	☐	☐
9. Bladder problems (difficulty in urinating, increased need to urinate, bladder incontinence)	☐	☐	☐	☐	☐
10. Dryness of vagina (sensation of dryness or burning in the vagina, difficulty with sexual intercourse)	☐	☐	☐	☐	☐
11. Joint and muscular discomfort (pain in the joints, rheumatoid complaints)	☐	☐	☐	☐	☐

Most people think that estradiol (estrogen) is the hormone of choice to treat the symptoms of menopause, but the results in Figure 2 confirm that testosterone is what you need.

Figure 2

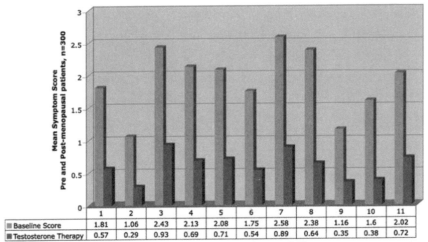

	1	2	3	4	5	6	7	8	9	10	11
Baseline Score	1.81	1.06	2.43	2.13	2.08	1.75	2.58	2.38	1.16	1.6	2.02
Testosterone Therapy	0.57	0.29	0.93	0.69	0.71	0.54	0.89	0.64	0.35	0.38	0.72

MRS Symptom Category, 1-11

In each column, the bars on the left represent the severity of symptoms before testosterone was given. Those are the baseline scores. The bars on the right represent the severity of symptoms three months after testosterone was given.

So, for example, column #1 corresponds to question #1: hot flashes and sweating. Before treatment, hot flashes and sweating had a score of 1.81—mild to moderate. After treatment, hot flashes and sweating received a score of 0.57—not completely gone but now milder than mild.

The interesting thing about this questionnaire is when you optimize testosterone levels to treat these symptoms, in every category on the questionnaire, you'll see that symptoms improved.

Here's the point: most everything you read about testosterone in women seems to skip the first forty years of a woman's life and focuses on helping her get her sex drive back. That's important and a very valid reason to optimize your testosterone levels! But testosterone is a valuable solution because it may also:

- Extinguish night sweats
- Help you sleep better
- Help you feel better
- Help you feel like you again
- Lift your mood
- Banish inner tension
- Boost your energy
- Boost your memory
- Boost your concentration
- Get rid of brain fog
- Help with bladder issues
- Reduce joint pain
- Improve vaginal dryness and discomfort
- Help you lose weight

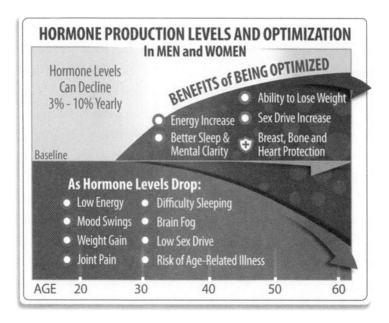

Signs of testosterone deficiency sneaking up on you.

At the same time as all these loud symptoms are making themselves known and making you miserable, something else has been silently going on. Without adequate levels of testosterone, you're at increased risk of:

- Alzheimer's disease
- Cardiovascular disease
- Osteoporosis-related fractures
- Diabetes
- Sarcopenia (the degenerative loss of skeletal muscle mass, quality, and strength that makes you frail and makes a broken hip a death knell)
- Breast cancer

I cover all of these health concerns in separate chapters, but I mention them here because there's more going on during menopause than most women realize. Sure, you may be able to handle some hot flashes or even getting up four times a night to head to the bathroom. But the silent degeneration of your health and vitality and the accumulation of damage in your blood vessels, brain, bones, and joints merit a serious conversation.

Studies confirm the importance of testosterone.

Many people say, "Well, there are just no studies on women to show that testosterone is better or worse or anything," but indeed there are. In fact, there was a double-blind, randomized, controlled trial in 1985 where Sherwin looked at estrogen and testosterone, estrogen alone, testosterone alone, and a placebo. The worst were estrogen alone and the placebo.

Testosterone was found to be superior for energy, well-being, somatic (physical) complaints, and psychological symptoms.

CASE HISTORY FROM A PRACTITIONER
Ruthann Rees, MD, Columbus, Georgia

L. D. is a forty-eight-year-old gravida 3 para 3 white female with a history of stage 0 intraductal carcinoma in situ found serendipitously at the time of a reduction mammoplasty many years ago. Before her breast reduction, her mammograms were normal. Because of her mother's history of colon cancer, she decided to undergo a prophylactic bilateral mastectomy with immediate reconstruction. L. D. had BRCA and Colaris gene testing and was negative.

She came to discuss menopausal symptoms she had been experiencing for many years. Her symptoms of vaginal atrophy were so severe that she had not been able to have sex for over a year. She had daily hot flashes, night sweats, difficulty sleeping, and fatigue. Her prior gynecologist had refused even to discuss HRT.

After an extensive discussion of her personal history of breast cancer, she decided to try testosterone therapy. She started on testosterone hormone optimization. At her six-week follow-up, she was elated with the vast improvement she experienced in relief of menopausal symptoms, especially with her sexual relations with her husband. She felt they were able to reconnect now on a physical and emotional level like they had not done in years. She reports this has saved her marriage.

"Age Healthier, Live Happier."

Look, I can't promise you an anti-aging solution. That phrase is silly. What I am saying is that when you optimize your testosterone, you can age healthier, keep your vitality, and live happier. Looking at Table X below, it is clear the benefits reach far beyond just improving your sex drive.

POSITIVE EFFECTS OF BIOIDENTICAL TESTOSTERONE IN WOMEN

- Enhance libido
- Heart protection
- Lower cholesterol/LDL
- Increased HDL
- Increased energy
- Enhanced sleep
- Feeling of overall well-being
- Reducing body fat
- Stronger bones and muscles
- Depression relief
- Reduced "brain fog"

MINIMAL SIDE EFFECTS

A Little History about Testosterone—the Elixir of Life

Early in the 1930s, Leopold Ruzicka, a perfume manufacturer and scientist awarded the Nobel Prize in chemistry, synthesized testosterone for the very first time. This was amazing because within two years of its being synthesized, it was actually injected into people. Very few drugs have ever been synthesized and then put into people in such a short timeframe.

Testosterone for women was pioneered by Robert B. Greenblatt, MD, in 1949. Appointed as the chair of the inaugural department of endocrinology at the Medical College of Georgia, Greenblatt developed the testosterone pellet and traveled all over the country treating women in menopause and teaching other physicians how to use testosterone and estradiol pellets to optimize their hormones.

There was such strong support for testosterone supplementation. There was great data, and, as you might imagine, patients experienced greater vitality and a better quality of life. That's because testosterone actually delivers relief from more symptoms of menopause than does estrogen.

That makes testosterone the most important hormone for women in every decade of life. Yet even to this day, there's no FDA-approved product for you.

3

TESTOSTERONE AND YOUR HEART

Is testosterone going to give me a heart attack?

JLC is an eighty-four-year-old female who, a few years ago, was suffering shortness of breath and difficulty doing her daily activities. After a visit to her cardiologist, she scheduled a cardiac stress test. She did poorly, as one would expect. She then had an echocardiogram to see how much blood was being pumped after the heart filled with oxygen-rich blood. (This is called the ejection fraction; a normal ejection fraction is 50 to 65 percent.) Her physician was disappointed that only 36 percent of this blood was being pushed out to her brain and other vital organs. She was hospitalized. A plethora of medications were started, all of which seemed to reduce the somewhat limited quality of life she had. Blood pressure medications reduced her blood pressure, causing extreme dizziness. Diuretics also caused dizziness to the point where she could not ambulate down the halls from her hospital room. She had been on statins before with extreme fatigue and muscle aches. No one thought to check her hormones because hormones are "dangerous" at her age, or so she was told. Once she had her testosterone optimized and no other medications added, her heart increased its ability to pump oxygen-rich blood by 30 percent. She went home and went off the medications she found unnecessary and was able to begin walking her dog for three, then four, then more blocks daily.

One Day at a Time was a television sitcom that ran between 1975 and 1984. It starred Bonnie Franklin as a single mom, Ann, raising two daughters. The show was funny and realistic, and, while I don't remember many episodes, I have never forgotten the December 1979 episode where Ann suffered a heart attack.

Now, why would that stick in my mind all these years? Because back then, the idea of a middle-aged woman having a heart attack seemed unbelievable. Men had heart attacks, not women!

Even now, when most people think "heart," they think "men." But here's the truth: cardiovascular disease (CVD) is the number-one killer of women in the United States.

Most women and their physicians don't realize that one in seven women dies from CVD before reaching menopause. Acute myocardial infarction (heart attack) in women younger than fifty-five years of age is increasing, not decreasing. In fact, CVD was responsible for killing 299,578 women in 2017—or about one in every five female deaths. For postmenopausal women, that number rises to one in three, two-thirds of whom had no previous symptoms.

Why are so many women dying from CVD?

The medical community is stuck in 1979. Forty-five percent of women are unaware that CVD is the number-one cause of death in women. Only 22 percent of primary care practitioners and 42 percent of cardiologists have sufficient knowledge to estimate risk of CVD. Only one-third of participants in cardiovascular clinical trials are female. Even the mice in animal studies are male. Although causes, symptoms, and outcomes of women's heart attacks are different than men's, that fact has been overlooked by the scientific community until quite recently.

Heart disease is silently ticking away.

Here's what I'd like you to know about your heart and CVD: atherosclerosis is the most common form of CVD. The term *atherosclerosis* comes from two Greek words: *athero* (paste, gruel) and *sclerosis* (hardness).

Arteries carry blood from your heart to the rest of your body. They're lined with a thin layer of cells—the endothelium—which is an organ that keeps your arteries smooth, allowing blood to flow freely, and is responsible for maintaining approximately sixty thousand miles of blood vessels in your body.

Atherosclerosis starts when the lining of your blood vessels becomes damaged. This damage occurs from inflammation caused by diet, medications, and medical conditions like diabetes. Inflammation leads to plaque formation.

This has been going on since you were a child.

Can you believe that men and women begin developing fatty deposits in their blood vessels as early as childhood?

Although age is the strongest risk factor for CVD, studies have shown that atherosclerosis begins early in life. The Pathobiological Determinants of Atherosclerosis in Youth (PDAY) study collected arteries, blood, other tissue, and data from three thousand persons fifteen to thirty-four years of age who died from external causes between 1987 and 1994. The PDAY study confirmed the origin of atherosclerosis (CVD) in childhood.

Plaques are made up of cholesterol, fatty deposits, cellular waste products, calcium, and fibrin (a clotting material in your blood). Sometimes plaques calcify and become hardened plaques, but often they remain soft and unstable, ready to be unroofed by additional inflammation. These plaques then allow your platelets to adhere, narrowing your blood vessels and reducing blood flow and necessary oxygen to your heart muscle. As plaque accumulates, it narrows your heart's arteries and gradually starves your heart muscle of the high level of oxygenated blood it needs to function properly. A lack of adequate blood supply to the heart typically produces symptoms that range from angina and unstable angina to heart attack or sudden death.

But menopause triggers rising levels of LDL cholesterol (which is often referred to as "the bad cholesterol"). Menopause also is a time when women's blood pressure is typically on the rise. Inflammatory mediators are increasing and worsening your risk of CVD and heart attack. Moreover, the lining of your blood vessels is under daily attack due to your unhealthy eating habits and inflammatory cells.

So if men and women are silently accumulating plaque at about the same rate over forty-plus years, why does a women's risk of CVD spike so high and more women than men suddenly drop dead from a heart attack or stroke at menopause?

If you remember from the chapter "Testosterone and Menopause," your testosterone starts declining in your third decade of life, and by age forty, you've lost 50 percent of your testosterone production. Production from your adrenal glands also declines, and women who have undergone bilateral oophorectomy experience a 50 percent further reduction in testosterone levels.

Studies have shown that women who have low testosterone have a higher number of plaques forming. They have more inflammation.

As your testosterone levels plummet, your immune system stops regulating inflammation; instead, inflammation increases in many areas of your body, including your coronary arteries.

A study conducted in 2011 at Frederich Schiller University of Jena determined that a woman's immune system produces nearly twice as many pro-inflammatory substances than that of men. Uncontrolled pro-inflammatory substances in your cells make disease worse, keep the fires of inflammation burning, and cause pain.

So why are your immune cells stoking the fires of inflammation? Low levels of testosterone.

When the women's immune system cells were treated with testosterone, inflammation was reduced. The lining of your blood vessels are allowed to then heal, and plaques are reduced.

In addition, women have a greater propensity toward obesity, insulin resistance, and diabetes—all risk factors for CVD. It appears that physicians have always assumed that estradiol was the protective hormone for women. Well, it is protective, but premenopausal women low on testosterone are suffering damage to their heart and, in many cases, heart attacks. Once again, that's why testosterone matters . . . more!

In addition, during menopause, your LDL (bad) cholesterol levels rise sharply, while your HDL (good) cholesterol levels decline.

So we have a trinity of events happening simultaneously—low testosterone + uncontrolled inflammation + increased LDL cholesterol—that are all triggered by a singular event: menopause.

As your testosterone levels plummet, dominant levels of estrogen increase your cardiovascular risk.

In April 2010, a study published in *The Journal of Clinical Endocrinology & Metabolism* evaluated the role that natural sex hormone levels play in CVD. It concluded that low androgen levels (testosterone) increase the risk of CVD in men and women. In addition, high local aromatase activity converting testosterone to estrogen in the heart increases cardiovascular risk. In addition, high estrogen in women may increase inflammation as it does in men.

That boost in LDL cholesterol production during menopause is boosting your risk of CVD.

An excellent study published in the 2009 *Journal of the American College of Cardiology* asked the question "Are Changes in Cardiovascular Disease Risk Factors in Midlife Women Due to Chronological Aging or to the Menopausal Transition?"

The study sample included 1,054 African American, Hispanic, Japanese, Chinese, and Caucasian women aged forty-two to fifty-two years. The results showed significant increases in total cholesterol, LDL cholesterol, and apolipoprotein-B (Apo B) within one year before and after the final menstrual period. Elevated total cholesterol can mean that not only are your LDL cholesterol levels increasing, but so are your triglyceride levels—both putting you at higher risk of heart disease or stroke. Elevated levels of LDL cholesterol increase the production of plaque.

As your testosterone levels plummet, your heart finds it harder to pump effectively.

What I want all women to know is that testosterone optimization will increase blood flow to your heart. It will reduce the number of dangerous plaques in your heart. Testosterone will also reduce insulin resistance, lowering your chances of developing diabetes, which is another risk factor for heart disease. Testosterone optimization in women with testosterone deficiency reduces inflammation in your body, and this helps protect your heart from future blockages.

CASE HISTORY FROM A PRACTITIONER
Christina M. Bove, MD, FACC

Bove, a well-respected cardiologist, sent me this testimonial:

Several years ago, after almost two decades of practicing traditional cardiology, I began a new, more functional medicine approach to CVD. This started with a new focus on nutrition and diet, followed by the addition of bioidentical hormone replacement (BHRT) to my services in 2017. With this approach, I quickly found I was able to *prevent and reverse* disease rather than merely treat symptoms of disease. I have been able to get my patients off anti-hypertensives, statins, and diabetic medications while improving their overall health, functional capacity, and quality of life. As a cardiologist, my daily focus is on cardiovascular prevention, as well as treatment of established disease. As CVD is a disease of inflammation, I focus on metabolic markers, advanced cardiac inflammatory panels, CIMT (measures the thickness of the inner two layers of the carotid artery and alerts physicians to any thickening when patients are asymptomatic), and coronary calcium scores rather than traditional lipid panels to establish patients' cardiovascular risk and treatment protocols.

I have seen firsthand in my patients the reversal of metabolic syndrome, diabetes, obesity, abnormal body composition, abnormal inflammatory markers, and dyslipidemia. Clinical studies have shown improvements in atherosclerosis and beneficial changes in heart muscle structure and function on cardiovascular imaging in patients receiving BHRT. From a cardiovascular standpoint, the anti-inflammatory, vasodilatory, endothelial function, vascular remodeling, and atherosclerosis benefits of testosterone therapy are compelling. I believe that with proper screening and follow-up, women using non-oral bioidentical hormones may benefit not only with marked symptom improvement but reduction in atherosclerosis, CVD, and overall mortality.

When we ask, "What do we have to help reduce heart disease?" the pharmaceutical industry answers, "Statins!" But this is a classic case of perception versus reality. There are no studies supporting the use of statins in the primary prevention of heart disease in women.

So the answer to the question "Is testosterone going to give me a heart attack?" is "No!" Testosterone is going to help protect your heart and reduce your risk of CVD. In fact, an expert panel convened at the 2015 American Association of Clinical Endocrinologists Annual Scientific and Clinical Congress stated, "The potential benefits of testosterone replacement therapy (TRT) to treat low testosterone (low T) in both men and women substantially outweigh any risks." Bioidentical hormone replacement therapy can reduce your chances for a heart attack.

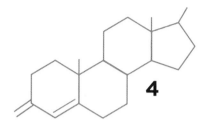

4

COGNITIVE DECLINE AND ALZHEIMER'S: IS THERE HOPE/HELP?

Why do women get Alzheimer's more than men?

Figure 3

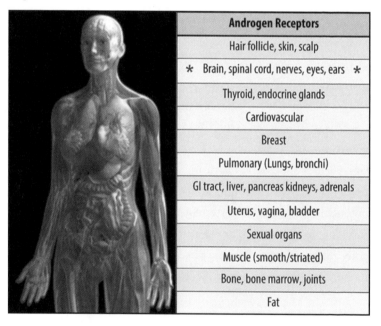

Androgen Receptors
Hair follicle, skin, scalp
* Brain, spinal cord, nerves, eyes, ears *
Thyroid, endocrine glands
Cardiovascular
Breast
Pulmonary (Lungs, bronchi)
GI tract, liver, pancreas kidneys, adrenals
Uterus, vagina, bladder
Sexual organs
Muscle (smooth/striated)
Bone, bone marrow, joints
Fat

Patient Testimonial

I was an anchor at a television station. My job was to interview, daily, the guests who brought relevant stories to our program. I studied the questions and the topics for conversation the afternoon before the interview and always felt prepared and excited to meet our "stars for a day." When I was in my mid-thirties, I began having trouble remembering the questions, the guest name, and the subject matter. I thought, I'm developing Alzheimer's disease like my mother. The drugs she took never brought her memory back. I was scared. I went to work with trepidation. One of my guests was Dr. Gary Donovitz. He said it might be my hormones. I was skeptical until Dr. D checked my labs. I was testosterone deficient. Once he optimized my testosterone, OMG, my brain fog and memory quickly reverted to the good ol' days. Thank you, Dr. D, for saving my job and my career.

At some point in your life, your brain is going to scare you because all those clichés about getting older start to come true: you can't remember where you left your keys; you walk into a room and have no idea why; and the parking lot is a sea of cars, and you can't recall where you parked yours.

They're most likely just memory slips and nothing to worry about. Yet your memory slips do serve to give you an unpleasant preview of what life with early-stage Alzheimer's might be like. I believe they're a valuable early warning system because—let's face it—who even thinks about their brain until something unusual happens? So let's talk about why it's important to pay attention as soon your brain sends a "can't find the darn keys" SOS.

What is Alzheimer's disease?

Alzheimer's disease (AD) is a form of dementia. Although all Alzheimer's patients have dementia, not all dementia patients have Alzheimer's disease. The Alzheimer's Association defines Alzheimer's disease as "a type of dementia that causes problems with memory, thinking and behavior. Symptoms usually develop slowly and get worse over time, becoming severe enough to interfere with daily tasks."

With Alzheimer's, deposits of β-amyloid (abnormal protein) plaques begin accumulating in the brain, eventually disrupting your normal brain function. As the deposits spread throughout your brain, brain cells begin dying (apoptosis), leading to further cognitive impairment. The nerves begin to entangle. Your brain shrinks. And, as you know, Alzheimer's is fatal.

"I have lost myself."

In 1906, the first person to be diagnosed with Alzheimer's disease was a woman named Auguste Deter. She was in her forties when she began suffering with loss of memory, delusions, and periodic vegetative states. She had trouble sleeping, would drag sheets across the house, and would scream for hours in the middle of the night. Mrs. Deter's husband, Karl, could not care for her—she did not even recognize him as her husband—and had her admitted to a mental institution in 1901. There, she was examined by Alois Alzheimer, MD, who identified:

- Untreatable paranoia
- Sleep disorder
- Memory disturbances
- Aggressiveness
- Crying
- Progressive confusion

When Alzheimer questioned her about the details of her life and she could not answer, glimmers of her awareness of her helplessness were revealed in one simple sentence: "I have lost myself."

She died in 1906. Alzheimer autopsied her brain and discovered β-amyloid plaques and neurofibrillary tangles—the hallmark of Alzheimer's disease.

Alzheimer's statistics are grim.

Every sixty-five seconds, someone in the United States develops Alzheimer's disease. Women have a higher incidence of Alzheimer's than men; out of the 5.8 million Americans who have it, 64 percent are women.

Once you're in your sixties, you are twice as likely to develop Alzheimer's than breast cancer and more than twice as likely to develop Alzheimer's than men. And when women develop it, Alzheimer's progresses twice as quickly, and their life span is shortened.

What are the signs of dementia/Alzheimer's?

Most age-related memory problems are not signs of dementia or Alzheimer's disease but evidence of a slowdown in the brain's processing speed that increases the time it takes to retrieve information. As we age, our ability to divide our attention among more than one task or bits of information also declines, which can interfere with storing new memories.

While you may be able to chalk up a few memory lapses to normal aging, there are some common warning signs of Alzheimer's disease. If you or someone you love is experiencing one or more of the following symptoms identified by Beverly Mertz, executive editor of *Harvard Women's Health Watch,* she recommends talking to your doctor.

Trouble remembering things. At first, only short-term memory may be affected, with long-term memory issues developing later. People may forget an appointment or the name of a new acquaintance. Many people complain of memory loss but can provide considerable detail regarding incidents of forgetfulness, such as where they were at the time. However, acknowledging memory loss only if asked and being unable to recall specific instances when they were unable to remember something can be a sign of dementia.

Mood or personality changes. It's natural for people to slow down as they age—perhaps they may not want to go to large gatherings if they can't hear or see well, or they may give up activities that have become physically challenging. However, changes in a person's basic disposition or temperament aren't normal and may be signs of dementia. For example, a person who was once social and outgoing may become withdrawn, or someone who was once cheerful may become stubborn, distrustful, angry, or sad. Depression also often accompanies Alzheimer's disease, causing such symptoms as loss of interest in a favorite hobby or activity, a change in appetite, insomnia or sleeping too much, lack of energy, and hopelessness.

Trouble completing ordinary tasks. Simple tasks that once caused no difficulty may become much more challenging. For example, forgetting how to use the oven, lock the door, or get dressed can be signs of Alzheimer's disease.

Difficulty expressing thoughts. One of the signs of Alzheimer's disease is having trouble with language. A person may try describing an object rather than using its name—for example, referring to the telephone as "the ringer" or "that thing I call people with." Reading or writing may also be impaired.

Impaired judgment. The individual might have trouble making decisions, solving problems, or planning. For example, he or she may no longer be able to balance a checkbook or pay bills.

Disorientation. We all know what it's like to be driving and momentarily forget where we're going. But getting lost in one's own neighborhood or losing track of the day or time can be two of the signs of dementia.

Unusual behavior. Wandering, becoming agitated, hiding things, wearing too few or too many clothes, becoming overly suspicious, engaging in unsafe behaviors, or using foul language may be signs of Alzheimer's disease, especially if a person hasn't behaved that way earlier.

The seeds of Alzheimer's were sown in your thirties and forties.

Alzheimer's begins with the development of mild cognitive impairment (MCI), which starts in your thirties and forties and takes fifteen to twenty years to develop. It affects men *and* women.

If both sexes are equally affected, then why is being female a major risk factor for developing late-onset Alzheimer's disease?

Are Alzheimer's and menopause connected?

It's menopause. In fact, brain-imaging studies demonstrate that forty- to sixty-year-old perimenopausal and postmenopausal women exhibit Alzheimer's characteristics such as decreased metabolic activity and an increase in the accumulation of β-amyloid deposits as compared to premenopausal women and age-matched men.

Clearly, there's a window of opportunity for intervention that would make a meaningful difference for thousands of women by combating the increased risk of Alzheimer's disease in women. But when you wait to start hormones until menopause, you lose that window of opportunity and instead allow years of cognitive decline and, at the same time, are literally starving your brain by withholding the hormones it needs to function and repair.

How do you protect against or combat Alzheimer's? Well, estrogen is one protective hormone, and testosterone is the other protective hormone.

But here's the catch: in the world of Alzheimer's research, the pink hormone, estrogen, is for girls, and the blue hormone, testosterone, is for boys. As a woman, here's why you'll age healthier and live happier when you start thinking "blue."

Testosterone reduces the production of β-amyloid plaque.

Increasing evidence indicates that testosterone, especially bioavailable testosterone, decreases with age; and, remember, there is a 50 percent decline by the time a woman reaches forty years of age. Alzheimer's disease is characterized by the age-related deposition of β-amyloid peptide aggregates in vulnerable brain regions. Multiple levels of evidence implicate a central role for β-amyloid in the development of Alzheimer's. Studies have shown that treatment with testosterone decreases the secretion of β-amyloid (Aβ peptides) from N2a cells and rat primary cerebrocortical neurons (specialized cells in the brain).

Several epidemiological studies have reported that estrogen replacement therapy protects against the development of Alzheimer's disease in postmenopausal women. In his book *How You and Your Doctor Can Fight Breast Cancer, Prostate Cancer, and Alzheimer's,* Ed Friedman explains how both estradiol and testosterone improve blood flow to your brain cells, how they both reduce β-amyloid, and how they both increase an enzyme to clean up β-amyloid that has already been deposited in your brain.

So if cognitive decline begins in your mid-thirties and β-amyloid deposition also begins then, and at that season of your life you have plenty of estrogen, what is causing the "brain fog"?

What is causing your brain to slow down? I believe it is the loss of testosterone. After losing testosterone for ten years, your brain is suffering one of the consequences of testosterone deficiency. Once again, that's why testosterone matters . . . more!

Testosterone improves memory and verbal learning in women.

In 2013, the results of the first large, placebo-controlled study of the effects of testosterone on mental skills in postmenopausal women who were not on estrogen therapy were presented at the Endocrine Society's ninety-fifth annual meeting.

Ninety-two healthy, postmenopausal women, ages fifty-five to sixty-five, received either testosterone or placebo. Both groups were tested before treatment, and both groups had similar cognitive function. After twenty-six weeks, the women who received testosterone therapy had a statistically significant and clinically meaningful improvement in verbal learning and memory.

Your brain was designed with testosterone in mind.

The parts of your brain that handle learning and memory are filled with receptors for testosterone.

CASE HISTORY FROM A PRACTITIONER
Brian Cox, MD, Austin, Texas

A sixty-nine-year-old female who underwent a left breast lumpectomy for breast cancer (1999) and who was diagnosed with mild, early Alzheimer's came to see me in January 2018 for HRT. She was on small amounts of testosterone by another provider. The patient's past medical history was also significant for osteoporosis, hyperlipidemia, type-2 diabetes, hypothyroidism, and rheumatoid arthritis.

Initial labs revealed total testosterone of 37. Her testosterone level showed she was clearly not optimized and, moreover, was symptomatic. She was started on testosterone 2 percent cream via daily topical application along with DIM 150 mg (a nutraceutical known to increase free testosterone). This was later increased to 4 percent testosterone cream due to low serum levels in April 2018. Finally, she achieved optimal levels with a serum level of 282 at the 4 percent dose.

The patient noted feeling better after a few months, and her husband said her mood was better as well. She was seen on September 26, 2019, for follow-up, and her husband stated they had recently seen her neurologist, who had tested her. He was amazed at her significant improvement and did not believe she had Alzheimer's but a milder form of dementia. What a relief for the patient and her husband!

Testosterone is going to help get rid of brain fog, help restore your mental edge, and protect you from Alzheimer's. The sooner you start, the better.

In fact, just imagine what Cox's patient's life might have been like if she had started optimizing her testosterone earlier! Timing is everything: the sooner you can replace what your body is deficient in, the less damage will accumulate in your body's organs.

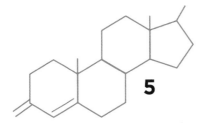

5

OSTEOPOROSIS:
CAN WE PREVENT THE BAD BREAK?

Protecting You from the Deadly Broken Hip

Figure 4

Androgen Receptors
Hair follicle, skin, scalp
Brain, spinal cord, nerves, eyes, ears
Thyroid, endocrine glands
Cardiovascular
Breast
Pulmonary (Lungs, bronchi)
GI tract, liver, pancreas kidneys, adrenals
Uterus, vagina, bladder
Sexual organs
Muscle (smooth/striated)
* Bone, bone marrow, joints *
Fat

Patient Testimonial

My mom had osteoporosis. My doctor said I could not take

hormones because of my history of breast cancer. She put me on a drug called Raloxifene, which she said would help build bone. OMG, the hot flashes were unbearable. I stopped the medication after three weeks. What I haven't told you is that my mom had a hip fracture at age seventy-eight. She passed away less than a year later from complications from the hip fracture, the doctors told me. I was frightened and felt like I was on a similar path in my life. My weak bones actually were causing me severe back pain, and I was losing height. I used to be five feet, five inches; now I was five feet, three and a half inches. My quality of life was diminishing. I found a doctor who said I should be on testosterone. He said it would build bone better than any other hormone replacement and was safe to take with my history of breast cancer. A year later, my DEXA bone scan improved by 11.2 percent. My QOL was so much better, and my back pain was markedly better. I was amazed to know that my life did not have to have the disastrous ending I experienced with my mom.

Like atherosclerosis, CVD, and Alzheimer's, osteoporosis is silent and sneaky. Often, there are no symptoms until the first fracture occurs. That's when you discover that your bones had been losing strength *for years.*

Osteoporosis is a disorder in which loss of bone strength leads to skeletal fractures. Fundamental pathogenetic mechanisms underlie this disorder, which include excessive bone resorption from the osteoclast, resulting in loss of bone mass, disruption of architecture, and failure to replace lost bone due to defects in bone formation from the osteoblast. In 1940, the American physician and endocrinologist Fuller Albright described postmenopausal osteoporosis and proposed that it was the consequence of impaired bone formation due to estrogen deficiency. Although estrogen deficiency is known to play a critical role in the development of osteoporosis, calcium, vitamin D, and vitamin K2 deficiencies and secondary hyperparathyroidism also contribute. Moreover, testosterone, the "bone builder," has been found to have an even more significant role. The rapid and continuous bone loss that occurs for several years after menopause must indicate an impaired bone formation response.

In younger individuals going through the pubertal growth spurt, even faster rates of bone resorption can be associated with an increase in bone mass. There are multiple mechanisms underlying the regulation of bone remodeling, and these involve not only the osteoblastic and osteoclastic cells but also other marrow cells. The interaction of estrogen, testosterone, and osteocalcin combined with local cytokines and growth factors all interplay in the continuum of the multifactorial process of bone remodeling.

Around the world, one in three women and one in five men aged fifty years and over are at risk of an osteoporotic fracture. In fact, an osteoporotic fracture is estimated to occur every three seconds.

The most common fractures occur at the hip, spine, and wrist. After a hip or vertebral (spine) fracture, direct and indirect mortality can be as high as 25 to 30 percent in the first year.

Osteoporosis, characterized by the loss of bone mass and strength that leads to fragility fractures, has probably existed throughout human history but only recently became a major clinical problem as human lifespan increased. Up until the 1930s, nearly half of women only survived until age fifty. After 1970, morbidity and mortality from infectious diseases were reduced, and long-term survival increased. In the early nineteenth century, Sir Astley Cooper, a distinguished English surgeon, noted "the lightness and softness that [bones] acquire in the more advanced stages of life" and that "this state of bone . . . favors much the production of fractures."

Why can bones become fragile and as full of holes as Swiss cheese? It's your hormones.

Your hormones are the reason your arms are the same length.

Estrogen and testosterone (androgen) are the hormones that influenced the size and shape of your skeleton and played an important role in your bone growth. After your birth, they were responsible for initiating and managing the process that made your long bones increase in length. Then, at the beginning of puberty, you experienced a growth spurt, again courtesy of testosterone and estrogen. At the end of puberty, they commanded bone growth to stop. Bone formation and the acquisition of bone-mineral density continued until you were about twenty-six years old, when you entered a maintenance phase of constant bone remodeling.

Your bones are like your heart.

Bones are living tissue and are made of living cells just like your kidneys, heart, and other organs. You were born with about three hundred soft bones. During childhood and adolescence, your soft bones grew and, by the end of puberty, had been replaced by hard bone. Some of your original three hundred bones eventually fused together, and you entered adulthood with a final adult skeleton consisting of 206 bones. In addition to providing support, attachment sites for your muscles, and protection for vulnerable internal organs, your bone also provides a home for bone marrow and acts as a reservoir for minerals.

Testosterone Assists the project manager in bone remodeling.

Bone remodeling is a highly complex process. Remember, bone is a live tissue and is continuously remodeling itself to maintain maximum bone-mineral density and to repair any small or large damage such as fractures. Remodeling is controlled jointly by estrogen and testosterone—except for one major difference.

Bone cells called osteoclasts break down old bone (resorption), and new bone is formed by bone cells called osteoblasts. But what controls the process? Bone cells called osteocytes are the project managers that coordinate the actions of osteoclasts and osteoblasts, maintaining the yin and yang of breakdown/resorption with growth/renewal.

Androgen receptors, the docking stations for testosterone, and estrogen receptors, the docking stations for estrogen, are both located on osteoblasts (the bone builders) and osteoclasts (the bone destroyers). But osteocytes, the project managers, only have androgen receptors. They need testosterone. That's why, again, testosterone matters . . . more!

In the Raisz study, women treated with conjugated equine estrogen (CEE) showed decreased serum markers of bone formation. In contrast, women treated with estrogen/androgen therapy showed significant increases in serum bone formation markers.

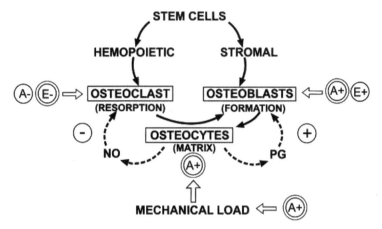

Figure 5

Bone remodeling, sex steroids, and mechanical loading, E, Estrogen; A, Androgen; NO, nictric oxide; +, stimulatory; -, inhibitory; PG, prostaglandin; double circle, primary activity; single circle, secondary activity. (From Smitt and Berger (1). Reprinted by permission of the publisher.)

Notelovitz, Androgen effects on bone and muscle. Fertil Steril 2002

Up until age forty, your bone remodeling happened without a hitch.

From approximately age twenty-six until age forty, you had plenty of testosterone to manage bone remodeling. But forty (on average) is the age when the bone cells responsible for breaking down bone in the remodeling process are no longer in sync with the bone cells responsible for producing new bone as a replacement. Bone loss begins outpacing the growth of new bone, and your bones begin to become porous, brittle, and prone to fracture. This process can be disrupted earlier in life if you are on birth control pills, which increase sex-hormone-binding globulin, a protein that binds your testosterone and reduces the amount of free testosterone. This immediately starts the reduction in your bone density and bone building.

Losing height may be your sign of reduced bone strength.

Davidson et al. have shown us a significant association between total testosterone and diminished vertebral bone mass. Lower androgen levels, reduced hip bone-mineral density (BMD), and an increase in hip fractures have also been noted. Lower bioavailable testosterone is correlated with loss of height.

Where did your project manager go?

As you may recall from an earlier chapter, by age forty, a woman has lost half of her testosterone production. Androgen production from the adrenal glands declines, and testosterone production from the ovary remains relatively intact after menopause. Adrenal secretion of androstenedione declines by 50 percent, resulting in a significant reduction in peripheral conversion of testosterone at menopause.

Losing strength is your body's SOS that you're losing bone.

Approximately 4 percent of muscle mass is lost during the first three years after menopause. You notice you're not as strong, and many older women begin falling. This is an SOS from your bones. The loss of muscle strength happens first and is then followed by the loss of bone mass.

Testosterone increases muscle mass and strength.

The results of a two-year study conducted by Morris Notelovitz, MD, PhD, published in *Obstetrics & Gynecology*, the official publication of the American College of Obstetricians and Gynecologists, concluded that testosterone "has a profound influence on the preservation of bone and on muscle mass and strength. The scientific rationale for androgen (testosterone) therapy is well founded."

Dr. Notelovitz's single-blind study treated women with either subcutaneous pellets of estrogen or subcutaneous pellets of estrogen + testosterone. Bone mass density increased in both groups, but the combination of estrogen + testosterone increased bone mineral density faster and to a greater degree.

Postmenopausal testosterone therapy increases lean tissue mass and decreases fat mass.

Another study measured the effect testosterone has on lean tissue mass and fat mass. A double-blind, randomized study evaluated body composition in two groups: one group was treated with estrogen, and a second group was treated with estrogen + testosterone. The estrogen + testosterone group had a significant increase in lean tissue mass and a comparable improvement in lower body muscle strength. In addition, it noted that the changes in the estrogen + testosterone group were significantly greater than those in the estrogen-only group.

Testosterone = bone builder.

J. W. W. Studd, MD, conducted a one-year study comparing the effect on bone density after changing from oral estrogen therapy to subcutaneous pellet estrogen + testosterone therapy. Twenty women who were receiving long-term estrogen replacement participated. Ten women changed to subcutaneous estrogen + testosterone pellets while ten continued with oral estrogen.

Published in the *British Journal of Obstetrics and Gynaecology*, the study results revealed that bone density increased significantly—by 5.7 percent—at the spine and by 5.2 percent at the neck of the femur in those women who had changed to the subcutaneous pellets with testosterone. No change or improvement was noted in the ten women who had continued with oral estrogen-only therapy.

The results of a second study conducted by Studd published in the *American Journal of Obstetrics & Gynecology*, revealed similar, exciting results. Twenty-three postmenopausal women with a median of two years past menopause (the range was one to 12 years) and a median age of fifty-two participated in this study. All women received subcutaneous pellets of both estrogen and testosterone. Bone density increased 8.3 percent at the spine and 2.8 percent at the neck of the femur. Oral estrogen replacement therapy like Premarin®, Prempro®, Enjuvia®, or Duavee® will increase bone density 1 to 2 percent per year.

Testosterone is going to protect your bones. It's also going to improve your ability to move and stay active. And here's the bonus with that: keeping active may be tied to a lower risk of dementia.

Recently published in the journal *Neurology*, a study involving eight hundred Swedish women with an average age of forty-seven were followed for forty-four years. Women who were physically active were 52 percent less likely to develop dementia and 56 percent less likely to develop mixed dementia than the women who were inactive.

CASE HISTORY FROM A PRACTITIONER
G. DeAn Strobel, MD, FACOG

I am a board-certified OB/GYN and practice in an area with a large geriatric population. When I first started my practice in 1999, I was overwhelmed with the number of osteopenia and osteoporosis patients I encountered.

I became so intrigued with the spectrum of disease that I pursued certification with the International Society of Clinical Densitometry (ISCD). I purchased my first DEXA machine in 2002.

Once ISCD-certified, I began to appreciate the nuances of DEXA interpretation and began to discover many otherwise asymptomatic patients with osteoporosis-related fractures. From what I understand, I was the first gynecologist in the state approved to prescribe and use teriparatide for patients with severe osteoporosis. I have also used all the various bone medications including SERMs, bisphosphonates, PTH-analogs, and even calcitonin. I have followed patients with serial DEXA scans for many years.

When I was initially trained by Dr. Donovitz and learned that pellet therapy can increase bone mineral density by up to 8.3 percent per year, I was apprehensive. It wasn't until a year or so after I began to use the pellets in patients that I began to see such dramatic improvements in their bone density scans. I have had many patients who have had DEXA scans change from T-scores in the osteopenia range to normal range, and I even have had some who have had complete reversal of osteoporosis. I am now a true believer!

My prescription numbers for bisphosphonates and other osteoporosis medications have dramatically decreased, and my patients' results have dramatically increased since I started using bioidentical hormone pellets and hormone optimization in my practice.

Clinicians should also understand that we have sufficient tools today to assess fracture risk and prevent as well as treat osteoporosis. Adequate calcium and vitamin D intake and appropriate physical activity may not only increase peak bone mass but also slow bone loss and reduce fracture risk throughout life. In addition, improvements in diagnosis and therapy are important, and certainly the selective estrogen receptor modulators and monoclonal antibodies have shown great promise in some clinical studies. As we face the millions of women who suffer from osteoporosis and the sequelae from the disease, patients should be encouraged by our current knowledge and the ability to build strong bones throughout their lives. It is critical that we apply this knowledge, which means a more widespread utilization of testosterone in women to deal effectively with the increase in osteoporosis and fractures that is projected as our population ages.

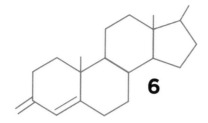

6

ENDING MUSCLE AND JOINT PAIN

Figure 6: Androgen Receptors in Females

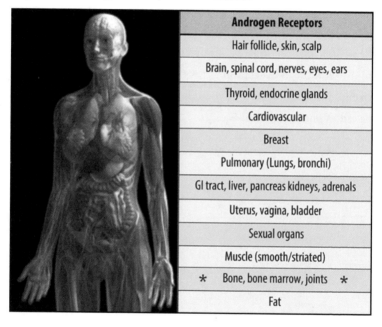

Androgen Receptors
Hair follicle, skin, scalp
Brain, spinal cord, nerves, eyes, ears
Thyroid, endocrine glands
Cardiovascular
Breast
Pulmonary (Lungs, bronchi)
GI tract, liver, pancreas kidneys, adrenals
Uterus, vagina, bladder
Sexual organs
Muscle (smooth/striated)
* Bone, bone marrow, joints *
Fat

Patient Testimonial

At a young age, while playing sports, we are told to ignore pain. Pain means you're pushing yourself; pain means you're getting better; pain means you're succeeding; pain isn't a thing you talk about. We are taught to push aside pain, and eventually we do. Pain: a word used in an entirety of different contexts. But for some, especially athletes, it means one thing: nonexistent.

Years later, along with several injuries in the rearview mirror, you don't notice the obnoxious pop your ankle makes every time you run or the shooting pain through your knee, reminding you of the meniscus tear you experienced a couple years prior; the dull ache in the shoulder from the fourteen times your shoulder dislocated when throwing home from center field or the radiating discomfort from the low back and hip region after diving for a ball, dislocating the hip and slipping a disc in the lower lumbar part of the spine; or the agonizing discomfort from the knee down through the ankle, known as shin splits/tendonitis of the IT bands from pounding the pavement, trying to qualify for a collegiate national track championship. We don't know a life without pain because pain becomes the new normal.

As the years go on, the training becomes more intense, practices go from two hours to five, expectations are heightened, and your entire mental and physical being is tested day in and day out. The cortisone injections and continuous flow of ibuprofen that started at age fifteen, along with the physical therapy and chiropractic care, just seemed to be a Band-Aid to make it through the next workout, next game, next practice, or next tryout.

When the day comes when we realize the pain isn't normal and wonder that maybe we shouldn't be hurting this much, we may seek treatment. For some, an underlying problem is introduced. A pain that is even further beneath the pain— whether it is genetic, brought on by a reoccurring injury, or simply developed on its own. One day, it hits you like a brick wall, and you realize the toll that your disease and your pain are taking on you. I always believed that both arthritis and chronic pain usually happen in older people. I was wrong. I was only twenty-five!

As a physiologist, through a process of trial and error, I eventually found a "medication" that works. After two children, fifteen-plus years of physical trauma, and multiple surgeries, my body had physically become dysfunctional, mentally exhausted, and emotionally drained. At age 33, I had hit rock bottom and finally got my hormones tested and found out that my total testosterone level was five. My testosterone was of a postmenopausal female and had completely been depleted.

On top of the chronic pain, I was also dealing with some depression, chronic fatigue, impaired memory, muscle atrophy, and suppressed libido. The clinic I worked for at the time had recently gotten trained to offer testosterone hormone pellet therapy, and, after doing tons of research, I had the provider pellet me. Game changer! Within a little over a week, the joint pain was the first symptom to subside, and I could get out of bed in the morning without doing the awkward roll to one side that I had done for almost ten years. The continuous, stabbing pain that had been radiating from my spine, through my hip, and down to my ankle had been alleviated, and I found myself again. It has changed my life, and I am so thankful for this amazing therapy I stumbled upon that gave me my life back.

When it comes to pain and pain management, men are "brave," and women are "emotional." That means your pain may not be addressed with the same seriousness and respect that men receive.

Women suffer chronic pain as they age.

Here's the thing (and you probably know this already from your own experiences): there's a long history of dismissing women's pain. Women in acute pain are left to suffer for longer in hospitals, they are more likely to be diagnosed with mental health problems (because they are "emotional"), even when clinical results show their pain is real, and they are consistently allocated less time than male patients by hospital staff due to men's complaints being perceived as more authoritative and important.

Why don't we know how to treat women's pain?

According to Amy Miller, PhD, president and CEO of the Society for Women's Health Research (SWHR), "Sex and gender bias has its roots in the way medical research was conducted for centuries—by simply assuming women's biology was the same as men's and excluding women from research. As recently as twenty-five years ago, women of reproductive age were actively excluded from most clinical trials." Similar to studies in cardiovascular health, even the animals used in pain studies have been male.

I guess there are far too many physicians and scientists who think that the human capable of growing a fetus internally and then, at the right time, pushing him/her into the world is exactly the same as the human who is not capable of such a miracle. That attitude never ceases to amaze me. As an OB/GYN for the past thirty-five years, I've treated thousands of women for many conditions, and I know without a doubt that your pain is different from your husband or brother's pain.

The link between menopause and chronic pain have been confirmed.

A newly published cross-sectional study of more than two hundred thousand national Veterans Health Administration medical and pharmacy records of women veterans aged forty-five to sixty-four revealed that the risk of conditions that cause or increase pain is highest in midlife women and women who are entering perimenopause or menopause.

Women are more likely than men to report chronic pain conditions such as back pain, fibromyalgia, arthritis, and osteoarthritis. Women with these conditions additionally report greater pain severity and pain-related disability than men.

The study confirmed that women with menopausal symptoms had nearly twice the chance of having chronic pain and multiple chronic pain diagnoses.

What's causing and/or increasing pain in perimenopause and menopause?

Low levels of testosterone. As I've mentioned previously, testosterone production in women comes from three sources: your ovaries, your adrenal glands, and then conversion from other circulating androgens in the bloodstream. Testosterone starts decreasing very early on, and by the fifth decade, by age forty, a woman has lost half of her testosterone production. Androgen production from the adrenal glands declines, and testosterone production from the ovary remains relatively intact after menopause. Adrenal secretion of androstenedione declines by 50 percent, resulting in a significant reduction in peripheral conversion of testosterone at menopause. And women who have undergone bilateral oophorectomy experience a 50 percent further reduction in testosterone levels.

As if that weren't enough, constant pain and pharmaceutical pain drugs are stealing what little testosterone you are able to produce.

Chronic pain steals your testosterone.

If you've dealt with pain or been with a loved one who is in pain, you know there is no greater stress to your body than pain.

Pain sends a fight-or-flight message to your hypothalamus-pituitary-adrenal system (HPA axis) that activates a release of adrenalin, cortisol, pregnenolone, and testosterone from your adrenal gland. You see the lion, and you run away fast. Once you're safe, your HPA axis returns to its normal production levels.

But nothing goes back to normal with constant pain. Pain itself can cause hyperarousal of the HPA axis, depleting patients of hormones such as cortisol and testosterone. Your HPA axis does its best to keep secreting cortisol and testosterone, but eventually your adrenal glands can't keep up, and they shut down. This is called adrenal exhaustion.

Opioids steal your testosterone.

It's well known that opioids have a suppressive effect on the production and secretion of hormones; the most common hormones suppressed are pregnenolone and testosterone. Patients on chronic opioid therapy have the highest prevalence of symptoms of testosterone insufficiency, which include muscle and joint pains.

Why testosterone must be a critical component of pain management for women.

It's difficult to find studies and data that specifically relate to testosterone and the management of pain in women. Most medical professionals are primarily interested in the sexual effects of testosterone. A new Consensus report by Susan Davis, MD, and her colleagues states that testosterone in women should only be used for hypoactive sexual dysphoric disorder. This group unfortunately overlooked the more experienced Consensus report that was published in 2020. This International Consensus group unanimously agreed on the multiple benefits of testosterone use in women. Frankly, that's one of the reasons I wrote this book. If testosterone is known to be an effective pain management solution, it's almost criminal to exclude women from the studies and benefits. Obviously, the benefits of testosterone in women are apparent throughout the body. What is lost in the recent controversies, however, is that the vast majority of testosterone is not prescribed to pain patients but rather to males and females for maintenance of libido, muscle mass, mood, and energy. Of course, these symptoms resonate with chronic pain patients, but testosterone has four additional critical properties in pain patients:

1. Protection and regeneration of damaged neural tissue;
2. Maintenance of opioid effectiveness so dosage can be minimized;
3. Prevention of opioid complications, including osteoporosis;
4. Analgesic effects in reducing pain.

In my clinical experience of training pain management physicians across the United States and in their testimonials reported back to me, a large percentage of their pain patients who start testosterone have witnessed these four benefits. Nearly 85 percent of chronic pain patients have testosterone deficiency. Testosterone's neuroprotective, neurogenic, and analgesic properties are underappreciated in the medical community. The only cases in which this would be contraindicated are patients with active cancer of the prostate, ovaries, and/or breast.

Testosterone improves most forms of chronic muscular pain: osteoarthritis and fibromyalgia.

Ten percent of men and 18 percent of women over the age of sixty have osteoarthritis. As predicted by the World Health Organization (WHO), it is now the fourth leading cause of disability. As we saw in the heart, there are progenitor cells in joints that can heal damaged tissue. These progenitor cells are stimulated by both estrogen and testosterone. In a large study in Korea in more than four thousand women, there was a reduction in osteoarthritis in those who maintained HRT for more than one year.

The incidence of fibromyalgia in postmenopausal women is between 6 and 7 percent. However, the mean age for the onset of symptoms is in the mid-forties, ahead of the onset of menopause. Symptoms of fibromyalgia include chronic fatigue, muscle pain, muscle wasting, and sleeplessness. These, you might recall, mimic those of testosterone deficiency. Non-steroidal anti-inflammatory drugs, opioids, and antidepressants all have been tried as therapies with limited success, the development of drug tolerance, and medication dependence. In addition, side effects like weight gain, gastrointestinal (GI) disturbances, and social dysfunction limit their usefulness.

Treatment with testosterone showed a dramatic improvement in symptoms without the side effects. Patients were screened with the fibromyalgia impact questionnaire and tender-point examination. Treatment with testosterone led to a dramatic improvement in symptoms, an improvement in the fibromyalgia impact questionnaire, and marked decrease in tender-point pain levels.

Throughout this book, we have read numerous physicians' testimonials. The following testimonial is especially memorable, for the treatment was for the physician herself. She was a forty-five-year-old Ivy League medical school professor who suffered from chronic fatigue, muscle pain, and insomnia. All of her medications were of minimal benefit and caused sexual dysfunction and weight gain. She surmised that testosterone was a muscle-building hormone and decided to be treated with testosterone HRT. The results were, as reported in a medical journal, both "immediate and enormous."

One of the more intriguing published studies explored the effect of hormone administration in transsexual patients.

Male-to-female transsexuals (MtF) are administered estrogens and anti-androgens (anti-testosterone), while female-to-male transsexuals (FtM) are administered androgens (testosterone) during the process of sex reassignment. Questionnaires dealing with pain were given to both MtF and FtM transsexuals undergoing hormone treatment for sex reassignment for at least one year. Forty-seven MtF and twenty-six FtM completed the questionnaires.

Approximately one-third of the MtF subjects developed chronic pain during their treatment with estrogen and androgens. Even those who did not develop chronic pain reported a decreased tolerance to painful events and an enhanced sensitivity to thermal stimuli (both warm and cold).

However, of those FtM patients who had chronic pain before the start of treatment, more than half improved after starting testosterone treatment, reporting reduced numbers of painful episodes and shorter lengths of those that did occur.

How are women treated for chronic pain? The answer is proving to be deadly.

A recent *Washington Post* article reviewed a database maintained by the Drug Enforcement Administration (DEA) that tracks the path of every pain pill sold in the United States and revealed that America's largest drug companies saturated the country with 76 billion oxycodone and hydrocodone pain pills from 2006 through 2012 as the nation's deadliest drug epidemic spun out of control.

According to the Centers for Disease Control and Prevention (CDC), from 1999 to 2010, the largest percentage changes in the rates of overall drug overdose deaths were among women in the age groups forty-five to fifty-four years and fifty-five to sixty-four years. Synthetic opioid-related deaths increased 1,643 percent between 1999 and 2017 among women aged thirty to sixty-four years, with the largest increases among those aged fifty-five to sixty-four and prescription-opioid-related deaths increased 485 percent for the same time period and age ranges.

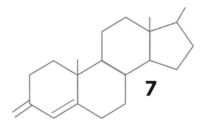

7

BREAST CANCER: DOES PREVENTION START WITH TESTOSTERONE?

Will testosterone give me breast cancer?

Figure 7

Androgen Receptors
Hair follicle, skin, scalp
Brain, spinal cord, nerves, eyes, ears
Thyroid, endocrine glands
Cardiovascular
Breast
Pulmonary (Lungs, bronchi)
GI tract, liver, pancreas kidneys, adrenals
Uterus, vagina, bladder
Sexual organs
Muscle (smooth/striated)
* Bone, bone marrow, joints *
Fat

Patient Testimonial

Shortly after my fortieth birthday, my life changed forever when, during a routine GYN visit, a lump was discovered in my left breast. In the end, I was diagnosed with stage-2 ER/ PR invasive ductal carcinoma. To translate, I had estrogen-receptive, progesterone-receptive cancer in the ducts of my breast, and several lymph nodes tested positive for cancer as well. I underwent the standard treatment after surgery: aggressive chemotherapy and radiation to my chest and armpit. The chemo left me on the far side of menopause: basically, they chemically induced menopause, and I endured hot flashes, night sweats, weight fluctuations, and all of the other "fun" symptoms of menopause . . . I just did it all in a condensed period of time.

To top off the chemo and radiation treatments, I was placed on Tamoxifen for two years as adjunct therapy. The complete fatigue I felt after all of the treatments and surgeries and this new medication left me feeling like a totally different person. I went from a healthy (I thought), happy professional with my own business to a fat, tired "old woman" with aches in every joint, especially my feet. No more heels for me—I was shopping for the dreaded comfortable walking shoe.

I struggled to regain my life for the next couple of years. Then my husband discovered bioidentical testosterone pellet therapy and was thrilled with his results. While I was truly happy for him and his newfound energy, inside I was despondent because I believed I would never "be allowed" hormone therapy because of my diagnosis. Thankfully, I was wrong! During a visit with my oncologist, I asked him about HRT and about bioidentical hormone pellets. At this point, I was three years from my last treatment. My doctor happily told me that I could indeed have testosterone but no estrogen or progesterone hormones. Within the week, I was at my nurse practitioner's office getting blood drawn. Soon after receiving my results, I was scheduled for pellets because my testosterone level was almost zero.

About two weeks after my first pellet treatment, I noticed that my feet weren't killing me all the time. Hmm. Then I noticed my energy level was increasing. No longer did I come home from work and put my feet up and pray the family was good with cereal for dinner! To my amazement, about a month in, I had enough energy for a whole-house deep clean. Imagine, with three teenage boys in the house, what that entailed! Somehow I even managed to make dinner on top of all that housework. This was the beginning of my journey to reclaim myself—and not just my energy level. I lost weight and regained some of the confidence I'd lost after surgery.

At the five-year anniversary of my last treatment, my oncologist released me from his care. He pronounced me cured and told me to go have a wonderful life. He told me, "Whatever you're doing, keep doing it. Your bloodwork has never looked better!" So in addition to supplements and management of my thyroid disease, the full component of bioidentical hormones really, truly gave me my life back—oh, and gave my husband his wife back!

—AR

In my practice and when I'm speaking around the world about testosterone for women, I often hear the same objection: I don't want to take hormones because I don't want to get breast cancer.

What they're saying is, "If I don't take hormones, then I won't get breast cancer." And that's just not true. The opposite is true. Your best protection may be testosterone.

This chapter is so important because there's new information that is already erasing all the old, outdated assumptions and replacing them with significant data not only to help protect you from breast cancer but to help improve your life and continue protecting you after a breast cancer diagnosis. The benefits of testosterone optimization are both exciting and life-changing to women in terms of healthcare.

Breast Cancer Myths

Breast cancer is one of the greatest health fears of women. In the United States, 240,000 women will develop breast cancer annually, and forty thousand will succumb to the disease.

Additionally, there were an estimated 63,960 cases of DCIS (localized breast cancer that has not invaded the surrounding tissue) in the United States in 2018. As you may know, DCIS is sometimes referred to as stage zero cancer. It means that there are abnormal cells that have not moved or spread from the breast milk duct in which they first developed. This is the most common type of noninvasive breast cancer.

Not surprisingly, for many women, magazine articles are a key source of information on breast cancer, but those articles are misleading not only in their assumptions but in the information they choose to include and exclude. This is how myths—and in the case of breast cancer, dangerous myths—are born.

MYTH: If I don't have a family history of breast cancer, I won't get cancer.

Breast cancer is often thought of as an inherited disease, but only about 5 to 10 percent of breast cancers are believed to be hereditary. The vast majority of people who get breast cancer have no family history. *In fact, the greatest risk factors are being a woman and growing older.*

MYTH: If I maintain a healthy weight, exercise regularly, eat healthily, and limit alcohol, I don't have to worry about breast cancer.

All of these behaviors can help lower your risk, but they can't guarantee you'll never get it.

MYTH: Annual mammograms guarantee that breast cancer will be found early.

An annual mammogram is the best tool we have for early detection, but it doesn't always find breast cancer at an early stage. Nevertheless, medical practitioners should be recommending mammograms starting by the age of fifty and continuing annually or biennially until the age of seventy-five if the patient is of average risk.

MYTH: Breast cancer always causes a lump you can feel.

As breast cancer is first developing, there might not be a discernable lump that can be felt during a self-exam. That is why the American Cancer Society reported in 2015 that it no longer recommends clinical breast exams, and the US Preventive Services Task Force reported the same in 2016. Get a mammogram.

Is testosterone the answer?

The median age of diagnosis of breast cancer for women in the United States is sixty-two, corresponding with the fact that, by that age, women have lost more than half of their testosterone production. We know testosterone is protective to the breast tissue.

A review of the history of androgen (testosterone) therapy reveals that testosterone and dihydrotestosterone were used successfully to treat breast cancer in the 1940s and 1950s. Unfortunately, inaccurate dosing not individualized to the patient led to masculinizing side effects. Now, decades later, the discovery of tamoxifen and aromatase inhibitors are thought to be better alternatives for the commercialization of breast cancer therapy with little thought being given to breast cancer prevention.

Surprisingly, the androgen receptor is the most widely expressed nuclear hormone receptor in the breast. The intracellular androgen receptor is present in 77 percent of breast cancer tumors. In luminal A tumors, 91 percent have the androgen receptor, while it appears in 68 percent of luminal B tumors and 59 percent expression in HER2 subtype tumors. Studies show an inverse relationship between tumors that possess the androgen receptor and the size, grade, and lymph-node status. On the contrary, tumors lacking an intracellular androgen receptor are mostly found to be grade 3 (fast-growing, poorly differentiated cells).

Most postmenopausal breast cancers are estrogen-receptor positive, and 75 percent of these tumors are androgen-receptor positive, allowing for us to increase apoptosis (cancer cell death) and decrease cellular proliferation (cell proliferation, or growth, is increased in tumors). In addition, cancers with the androgen-receptor expression have improved overall survival and disease-free survival. Not only is the androgen receptor associated with smaller tumors that are less aggressive and lower grade, but it has been shown to be associated with lower risk of recurrence. The androgen receptor is also an excellent predictor of therapeutic response to tamoxifen. In patients who are androgen-receptor negative, the response to tamoxifen is worse.

A study specifically looking at triple-negative breast cancer and the androgen receptor showed that the androgen-receptor expression, when present, reduces recurrence and the incidence of death. In estrogen-receptor negative (Er-), HER2-positive breast cancers, markers of proliferation like Ki-67 and carbonic anhydrate are lower if there are androgen receptors expressed, which is also associated with longer disease-free survival (DFS) and overall survival (OS). Impressively, 59 percent of triple-negative breast cancers are androgen-receptor positive and, therefore, a target-rich environment for testosterone optimization.

Taking testosterone optimization and breast cancer therapy one step further, if the tumor cells have androgen-synthesizing enzymes (i.e., capable of making testosterone and dihydrotestosterone intracellularly) and androgen-receptor expression, then proliferation markers as described above are negatively correlated, and survival is shown to be better.

A 10-year study conducted by Rebecca Glaser, MD, was undertaken to investigate the effect of long-term testosterone therapy on the incidence of breast cancer. Results were published in February 2019. A total of 1,267 pre- and postmenopausal women were enrolled in the study from March 2008 to 2013. They were treated with either subcutaneous testosterone implants (T) or subcutaneous implants with a combination of testosterone and anastrozole (T+A). The long-term therapy with T or T+A reduced the incidence of breast cancer by 59 percent during active therapy, which continued up to one year following the last implant.

Dr. Glaser conducted another study to determine the effect of testosterone, combined with anastrozole, on a hormone-receptor-positive, infiltrating ductal carcinoma. Three subcutaneous implants, each containing 60 mg of testosterone and 4 mg of anastrozole, were placed around a 2.4 cm tumor located in the left breast. By day forty-six, there was a sevenfold reduction in tumor volume and, by week thirteen, a documented twelvefold reduction in tumor volume. This novel therapy may prove to be a new approach to local and systemic therapies for breast cancer and has the potential to be used to reduce tumor volume, allowing for less surgical intervention.

In addition, I have just completed a ten-year retrospective review of more than 8,000 patients using testosterone and testosterone with estradiol delivered by sub-cutaneous pellets. This could be the largest review ever completed to better understand the prevention of breast cancer. The preliminary results showed a more than 70 perccent reduction in the incidence of breast cancer from the placebo group of patients in the Women's Health Initiative.

CASE HISTORY FROM
A PROMINENT BREAST CANCER SURGEON
IN A LETTER SHE RECEIVED
FROM HER PATIENT

I feel compelled to tell my story in hopes to get this out more to help other women as it did me.

In 2013, I was diagnosed with breast cancer. I was told at that time I could no longer take estrogen. I had been on estrogen for more than ten years due to a hormone deficiency. At the time, I was concerned but more concerned over the breast cancer and what I was about to endure.

Once all the surgeries and treatments were over, I struggled for three years with extreme hot flashes, emotional turmoil, and was very close to being suicidal. I had gone to my family doctor and my gynecologist and cried over this numerous times. They would tell me there was nothing they could do but give me anti-depressants, which I was already taking. During my annual visit to my gynecologist in late 2016, she had asked if I was still seeing my breast surgeon. I told her I was not. She then asked if I would see a different doctor, and I told her I would. I thought maybe at that time I might have a chance with another doctor of finding relief for myself.

While visiting the new breast surgeon, I was in the same shape as I was with the others, crying and telling her I needed help or I was not going to make it much longer. She agreed and said she would get with my gynecologist and let them know it was okay for some kind of hormone therapy. It took awhile, but I pushed the issue and finally was referred to a doctor in Dayton due to I was not yet out five years from my breast cancer.

Now I am having testosterone pellets inserted, and it is the best thing that could have ever happened to me. I know that I would probably not be here today had I not received this treatment. I was in such bad shape and had pushed so many people out of my life with being so hateful, etc. I now have more energy than I ever had, no more hot flashes, and I have become a new person.

This needs to get out more, and doctors need to learn more about this. I went three years telling them I was suicidal and really needed help, and all I got from them was there was nothing they could do. I feel my life was not important enough to them to help me with this option that saved my life.

It appears that the fears of developing breast cancer associated with HRT could potentially be prevented by proper hormone optimization, especially with the inclusion of testosterone. For those women whose lives have been compromised by breast cancer, hormone optimization with testosterone may not only improve their quality of life but may also be the therapeutic answer to improving their overall survival and defeating the cancer.

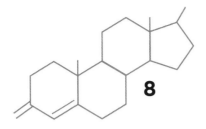

8

THYROID HORMONE: WORKS SYNERGISTICALLY WITH TESTOSTERONE IN HORMONE OPTIMIZATION

In 1656, Thomas Wharton named the gland located in the base of your neck the thyroid, after the shape of an ancient Grecian shield. It's also referred to as a butterfly shape. The thyroid gland releases hormones that regulate temperature, metabolism, cerebral function, and energy. A properly functioning thyroid increases fat breakdown, resulting in weight loss as well as lower cholesterol. The thyroid is also protective against CVD, cognitive impairment, fatigue, weight gain, and memory loss.

You never really noticed your thyroid, just as you don't notice your heart and bones, because it quietly and efficiently produced specific hormones that influenced every cell, tissue, and organ and regulated your vital body functions, including:

- breathing
- heart rate
- body weight
- muscle strength
- body temperature
- menstrual cycles

The American College of Obstetrics and Gynecology recommends screening for hypothyroidism after entering menopause. Unfortunately, subclinical hypothyroidism (a.k.a. type-2 hypothyroidism) affects 40 to 50 percent of the US population and begins in our teenage years. Thierry Hertoghe, MD, a Belgian endocrinologist, estimated the incidence to be as high as 80 percent in his country. As we meander through the seasons of our life, after our teenage years, many of our hormones begin a never-ending decline. One of the most important of these deteriorations is that which occurs with thyroid hormones.

Hypothyroidism, a disease in which the thyroid gland does not make enough thyroid hormone, is the second most common endocrine disorder among women. In addition to type-2 hypothyroidism, a very common autoimmune condition known as Hashimoto's thyroiditis affects one's thyroid homeostasis via the destruction of the thyroid gland. Hashimoto's affects 10 percent of the US population and is seven times more prevalent in women. It is one of the most common causes of hypothyroidism. More than 90 percent of patients with Hashimoto's have elevated thyroid peroxidase antibodies. These antibodies attack and destroy your thyroid gland. Hashimoto's comprises a vicious cycle of triggers (e.g., gluten, low iron, stress, leaky gut) and destruction, leading to depletion of nutrients and further thyroid compromise. Patients can fluctuate between being hypothyroid and hyperthyroid until eventually the thyroid gland is destroyed. The majority of patients with Hashimoto's have gluten intolerance, and the main protein in gluten is gliadin, which has a lot of similarity to proteins in the thyroid. Therefore, a diet with gluten often exacerbates the symptoms of Hashimoto's thyroiditis. In summary, patients with Hashimoto's need to have their triggers (gluten, stress, leaky gut) treated aggressively. A gluten-free diet and a good probiotic are mainstays of therapy and yet often neglected. They need their depletions (low iron, selenium, zinc) replaced.

Similar to what has been reported with testosterone, there are over two hundred symptoms related to thyroid deficiency. Many of these include but are not limited to cold hands and feet, thinning hair, weight gain, increase in body fat, decreased energy, loss of cognition, depression, menstrual irregularities, and a compromised gut motility. The long-term benefits of thyroid optimization have been reported to include an improvement in CVD, brain function, weight loss, and lipid profile. Optimization of T3 in obese patients with normal thyroid labs results in a statistically significant reduction in cardiovascular risk factors including lipid levels and insulin sensitization.

However, symptoms do not necessarily correlate with laboratory levels. Many uninformed practitioners and societies such as the American Thyroid Association and American Academy of Clinical Endocrinology have indicated no treatment is needed with a normal TSH level despite symptoms being present. Unfortunately, these guidelines result in the persistence of symptoms due to undertreated hypothyroidism and the utilization of other types of drug therapy to treat weight gain, cognitive decline, and other low-thyroid symptoms that result in poor quality of life for patients. Stated simply, TSH is a poor litmus test in gauging which patients need thyroid hormone optimization and determining if the patient has received adequate amounts of thyroid hormone.

Thyroid deficiency is often attributed to a decrease in hormone production by the thyroid gland. While this is one cause, two other significant causes should be considered. Thyroid deficiency can also be caused by decreased conversion of T4 to T3 as well as resistance at the receptor site, causing low-thyroid symptoms despite "normal" blood levels. These causes are similar to what is seen with testosterone deficiency and insulin resistance. Low T3 concentrations at the cellular level are a significant contributor to the symptoms of hypothyroidism. It is not the TSH or the T4 levels that are erroneously purported. The bottom line is that, as we age, we are less capable of converting T4 to the active hormone T3.

Unfortunately, one of the most prescribed medications is Synthroid, which is not an active hormone but rather a prohormone. Two studies clarify the point that as patients age, treating with T4 alone (e.g., Synthroid, levothyroxine) will never deliver optimal active thyroid hormone levels to your cells, and thereby mitochondrial function will be hampered. This means your cells will not have the energy to make the proteins your body needs. Therefore, how can you feel your best? How can the benefits of your testosterone hormone optimization be fully realized? The first study indicates that the majority of patients, at one time or another, suffer from stress, chronic inflammation, illness, obesity, insulin resistance, low testosterone, or dyslipidemia, resulting in disrupted transport of T4 into the cells of the body. Thus, the substrate (prohormone) needed to make T3 is reduced, resulting in an intracellular depletion of the active thyroid hormone T3. The second study clearly demonstrates that as we age, we are less capable of converting T4 to T3, and therefore treatment with T4 alone will not deliver optimal T3 levels in our vital organs.

In women, the leading cause of death is CVD. It is generally accepted that the euthyroid state (normal levels of thyroid hormones) is preferred for the cardiovascular system because both hyperthyroidism and hypothyroidism cause or accelerate disease processes. Hypothyroidism is known to be associated with atherosclerosis and ischemic heart diseases. To reduce the incidence of CVD, we must reduce inflammation and improve blood flow to the heart. Remember from the chapter on testosterone and the heart that the goal of hormone optimization is to improve blood flow and reduce inflammation. So the similarities of testosterone and thyroid hormone both in symptoms and beneficial outcomes to your body are quite comparable. Thyroid replacement therapy (TRT) and, more specifically, thyroid optimization reduce C-reactive protein (and other inflammatory substances that cause plaques in your blood vessels) and improve blood flow to your coronary arteries. In fact, it appears the lack of thyroid hormone leads to vaso-constriction of the arterioles. Therefore, low-active thyroid levels are associated with less blood flow to the heart muscle. The reality is that survival after acute myocardial infarction is greater if one's free T3 is optimal.

Also, just like with testosterone hormone optimization, myths have arisen surrounding thyroid hormone optimization.

Myth 1: Arrhythmias

Whereas patients with primary hypothyroidism can be prone to tachycardia (accelerated heart rate) and other arrhythmias of the heart, most patients treated for type-2 hypothyroidism do not experience heart arrhythmias. In fact, after thyroid optimization, they experience fewer serious arrhythmias.

Myth 2: Osteoporosis

Another fear of prescribing thyroid hormone is that patients will develop osteoporosis secondary to TSH suppression. This is a myth, far from reality, and is not supported by the evidence in the literature. Thyroid replacement therapy in premenopausal and postmenopausal women does not cause a reduction in BMD.

The litmus test for any interventional therapy, including optimization of all hormones, must start with improvement in clinical symptoms and encompass patient satisfaction while dually being cognizant of the side effects of the therapy. In a randomized double-blind crossover study comparing desiccated thyroid extract (DTE) to levothyroxine (L-T4), the majority of patients preferred DTE over L-T4. In all symptom categories, the desiccated thyroid was subjectively better, which will translate into better patient compliance and continuation rates. Overwhelming patient preference for DTE over L-T4 was also seen in the study comparing Armour thyroid to levothyroxine. In a large study involving twelve thousand patients, T4 replacement had the lowest patient satisfaction score. Participants reported better success with weight management, fatigue, memory and overall cognition, and mood swings using DTE. Two tenets to always remember in diagnosis and treatment of hypothyroidism from the legendary pioneer Broda Barnes, MD, are that TSH is a poor lab test and fails to diagnose a large percentage of patients with hypothyroidism, and, secondly, desiccated thyroid is more efficacious than Synthroid (levothyroxine).

In conclusion, thyroid management is imperative to optimization of hormone status and quality of life in patients. Low-thyroid symptoms are widespread and not always accurately reflected in lab results; therefore, if patients appear to be hypothyroid, treat them for their symptoms rather than focusing only on the lab tests. The incidence of secondary hypothyroidism is significant, and identification and treatment of this disease state are extremely important to actively managing patients' health status. The treatment of choice for most hypothyroid patients is DTE (desiccated thyroid extract including T4 and T3) rather than T4 alone as several patients have issues converting T4 in the peripheral tissue. Identification of Graves's disease and Hashimoto's thyroiditis is extremely important as it greatly influences the treatment plan. Untreated thyroid disease causes patients to remain in a substandard state of health and increases their risk factors. Practitioners should take this into consideration when developing individualized treatment plans for their patients.

There is no question that patients who have their thyroid hormone levels optimized coincidentally with their testosterone hormone levels will have better outcomes and improved quality of life.

CASE HISTORY FROM A PRACTITIONER

As with testosterone insufficiency, the patient's story tells us the reality if our therapy is working or not. Unfortunately, many practitioners have become dependent on lab tests and forgotten the most important question: "How does the patient feel?"

Dr. R had a thirty-five-year-old female come in with a diagnosis of hypothyroidism. She had been treated with Synthroid for five years (TSH 2.5, FT3 3.0). She had symptoms of weight gain, cold hands/feet, hair thinning, dry skin, and mild constipation.

The doctor changed her over to a desiccated thyroid (NP) that contained both T4 and the active thyroid hormone T3 and repeated her thyroid labs in eight weeks (TSH 0.5, FT3 3.8). Her active thyroid hormone was now in the optimal range. Importantly, her weight decreased by five pounds, she no longer had cold intolerance, and she was starting to see healthier hair as well as normal bowel function. She felt so much better overall.

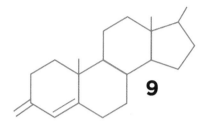

9

TESTOSTERONE AND SEXUAL HEALTH

Have we failed women?

I'm thirty-six years old, but I didn't have my first orgasm until a year ago. Before that, I couldn't help but think, This is sex? *What a disappointment.* I saved myself for my husband. *And I stuck to that—my hubby and I didn't have intercourse until we were married, when I was in my twenties.*

For me, it was another chore, and I felt nothing: There must be something more to this. *I know that he was frustrated, but I just got to the point that I didn't care, and neither did he, probably ruining our relationship.*

I knew there had to be an answer out there.

When I asked my gynecologist what I could do, he suggested masturbating. I thought, Are you kidding me? Nothing ever worked! Ever! *Child number two came along, and now here I was at age thirty-four, when my doctor did a lot of bloodwork on me and said I had very low testosterone levels—a significantly low level, in fact—and that I needed treatment.*

I started on testosterone-replacement therapy in 2017, and it fixed a plethora of things with my energy increasing, joint pain being alleviated, and libido working for the first time ever in my life. I actually felt what everyone else had been feeling all this time. With the medical aspect covered and a new relationship after a divorce of seven years, I stuck with treatment, and, at age thirty-five, I had my first-ever orgasm.

—MH

Sexuality is an important component of emotional and physical intimacy that most women desire to experience throughout their lives. In fact, female sexuality has been recognized by WHO not only as an important component of women's health but also as a basic human right.

Yet the prevalence of sexual dysfunction in postmenopausal women is estimated to be between 68 and 86.5 percent. Although there is a tendency to assume that women lose interest in sex after menopause, data from a European survey conducted with 1,805 postmenopausal women (aged fifty to sixty years) revealed that 71 percent reported that maintaining a sex life was important.

For men, the most common sexual problem is erectile dysfunction, but, among older women, sexual function diagnoses are more complex, and there is a vagueness about the diagnoses. Erectile dysfunction doesn't necessarily mean that a man's desire has decreased. In fact, it can be a warning sign of serious health issues that may eventually manifest as a stroke or heart attack. Yet for older women, the underlying medical reasons for sexual function difficulties receive less attention and treatment, even though common disorders related to sexual dysfunction and increasing age are, similar to men, also warning signs of serious health issues including CVD, diabetes, lower urinary tract symptoms, and depression.

Despite the existing knowledge about the importance older women give to staying sexually active, a study from Israel determined that "higher levels of ageist attitudes were found to be directed towards older women compared to older men. Older women are often afraid to involve physicians in their sexual problems and therefore choose to deal with these problems alone or to ignore them. When family physicians raise sexual issues, it usually occurs with older men, rather than with older women, despite studies which indicate a higher sexual dysfunction rate among older women."

Symptoms of Serious Sexual Health Issues

The 2013 Clarifying Vaginal Atrophy's Impact on Sex and Relationships (CLOSER) study surveyed 4,100 women representing the United Kingdom, Finland, Norway, Sweden, Denmark, Italy, France, Canada, and the United States and found that having sex less often (58 percent), less satisfying sex (49 percent), and putting off having sex (35 percent) were the main effects of vaginal dryness, soreness, itching, burning, and dyspareunia (pain). Fifty-five percent attributed intimacy avoidance to painful sex, and 46 percent indicated it was responsible for reduced sexual desire.

In the REal Women's VIews of Treatment Options for Menopausal Vaginal ChangEs (REVIVE) survey, 3,768 postmenopausal women between forty-five and seventy-five years old reported that their vaginal symptoms negatively affected enjoyment of sexual activity (59 percent), sleep (24 percent), and overall enjoyment of life (23 percent).

If sex is painful, if it makes you bleed or you're exhausted and have urinary tract infections (UTIs) all the time, you may want to enjoy sex, but you can't. We've got to address the underlying health reasons that are tamping out desire. With life expectancy for women reaching eighty-one years in the United States, the important goal is understanding and preserving sexual health for all women, and especially postmenopausal women, so women can control and enjoy a quality of life that they've determined is right for them.

The genitourinary syndrome of menopause (GSM) is a new term that describes an updated and more comprehensive understanding about the menopausal signs and symptoms associated with physical changes of the vulva, vagina, and lower urinary tract affecting sexual health. Moreover, GSM is chronic and progressive, increases in severity over time, and does not improve without treatment:

Table 2

Symptoms	Signs
Genital dryness	Decreased moisture
Decreased lubrication during sexual activity	Decreased elasticity
Discomfort or pain during sexual activity	Labia minora resorption
Post-coital bleeding	Pallor, erythema
Decreased arousal, orgasm, desire	Loss of vaginal rugae
Irritation, burning, or itching of the vulva or vagina	Tissue fragility, fissures, petechiae
Dysuria	Urethral eversion or prolapse
Urinary frequency and urgency	Loss of hymenal remnants
	Prominence of urethral meatus
	Introital retraction
	Recurrent urinary tract infections

Reprinted from "Genitourinary syndrome of menopause: new terminology for vulvovaginal atrophy from the International Society for the Study of Women's Sexual Health and the North American Menopause Society" [D.J. Portman and M. L. Gass, 2014; 21(10): 1063–1068, copyright 2014 by the North American Menopause Society]

Testosterone: The Regulator and Protector of Female Sexual Health

Menopause-related vaginal and bladder symptoms affect over 50 percent of midlife and older women. These symptoms have a marked impact on sexual functioning, daily activities, emotional well-being, body image, and interpersonal relations. In 2018, an International Society for the Study of Women's Sexual Health expert consensus panel review confirmed the value of androgens in the treatment of GSM.

The genitourinary syndrome of menopause affects the vaginal lining and the tissues in and about the bladder, all of which are both androgen- and estrogen-dependent. In addition, the clitoris, opening to the vagina (vestibule), vestibular glands, urethra, anterior vaginal wall, periurethral tissue, and pelvic floor respond well to androgen hormone therapy.

In double-blind, placebo-controlled clinical trials in naturally and surgically menopausal women, testosterone therapy resulted in statistically significant improvements in the number of satisfying sexual events, sexual desire, and sexual distress that were twofold greater than with placebo.

In a review of thirty-six trials with 8,480 women, approximately 95 percent of whom were postmenopausal, testosterone therapy significantly increased sexual function, including satisfactory sexual event frequency, sexual desire, pleasure, arousal, orgasm, and responsiveness, as well as increased self-image and reduced sexual concerns and distress. Once again, testosterone matters . . . more for postmenopausal women.

According to Susan Davis, MBBS, PhD, of Monash University in Australia, "Our results suggest it is time to develop testosterone treatment tailored to postmenopausal women rather than treating them with higher concentrations formulated for men. Nearly a third of women experience low sexual desire at midlife, with associated distress, but no approved testosterone formulation or product exists for them in any country and there are no internationally agreed upon guidelines for testosterone use by women. Considering the benefits we found for women's sex lives and personal well-being, new guidelines and new formulations are urgently needed."

10

SYNTHETIC VERSUS BIOIDENTICAL TESTOSTERONE

What is the difference, and which has the best outcome?

Testosterone therapy for women is not an alternative medicine. It's an alternative to bad medicine. Optimizing testosterone levels in women is an advanced, time-tested HRT with studies over the past eighty years that confirm the benefits. Of note for all women is the fact that testosterone therapy was utilized to treat the symptoms of menopause prior to the introduction of estradiol.

There are two options available: synthetic and bioavailable. Which has the best outcome? Let's quickly discuss the differences.

Table 3

BIOIDENTICAL VS. SYNTHETIC TESTOSTERONE

Bioidentical Molecule	Synthetic Molecule
• Exact molecular structure of hormones that the body produces	• Different molecular structure than what body produces
• Made from soy or yams	• Made from animal parts or urine
• Testosterone	• Testosterone cypionate, enanthate, undecanoate

It's important to note that all forms of testosterone, whether bioidentical or synthetic, are created in laboratories using chemical means. A bioidentical hormone is the exact molecular structure of the hormone that the body naturally produces. Most of the bioidentical testosterone is made from soy or yams.

Testosterone

Synthetic testosterones have changed the molecular structure and it no longer chemically matches the hormone as naturally made by the body.

Testosterone Cyplonate   **Testosterone Enanthate**

Why would a pharmaceutical company want to modify a perfectly matching testosterone molecule? The first reason has to do with functionality—the ease with which a substance is successfully used by the body—which is directly tied to the route of delivery. The second is the fact that natural hormones cannot be patented. What's made in nature is not patentable. However, if a drug company chemically modifies a hormone's structure in a unique fashion or develops a new formulation/system for a unique delivery method of a hormone (the route of delivery), that company may apply for a patent for that drug. If their newly created drug is approved by the FDA and their patent is accepted, then they may solely profit from the drug's manufacture for a number of years before other companies can create generic or brand-name equivalents. These modified hormones will produce some expected beneficial effects, but they can also generate many unwanted adverse reactions.

Table 4

ROUTE OF ADMINISTRATION - TESTOSTERONE

	Oral	Transdermal / Vaginal	Injectable	Pellet
Testosterone	Striant (buccal) Methyltestosterone (S)	Androgel (B) Axiron (B) Androderm (B)	Cypionate (S) Enanthate (S) Undeconate (S)	Testopel (B) Compounded (B) Manufactured (B)

Why is the route of delivery so important?

Table 5

Oral
- 1st pass effect
- GI upset or nausea
- Daily administration
- Hepatotoxic (methyltestosterone)
- Testosterone itself given orally not effective
- Buccal/sublingual forms – must be dosed TID; very short half-life

Transdermal/vaginal/scrotal
- Skin irritation
- 45% of people do not absorb
- Have to administer daily or BID
- Blood levels vary
- **Possible transfer to others**

WHY DOES DELIVERY MATTER?

Injectable
- Weekly/biweekly administration
- Fluctuating levels ("roller coaster")
- Pain with injection
- Allergies to oil suspension
- Higher level of erythrocytosis & aromatization
- May increase platelet stickiness

Pellet
- More consistent blood levels over time
- Some pain with insertion
- Possibility of extrusion
- Activity restrictions after procedure

Testosterone is not stored by the body for future use, so to maintain healthy levels, it must be administered in timed intervals and in appropriate dosages.

Oral

Drugs that are taken orally (swallowed) are absorbed from the gastro-intestinal tract and pass via the portal vein into the liver. If bioidentical testosterone is given orally, a very large portion is metabolized during this first pass through the liver, and therefore it cannot become bio-available to do its work in the body. Oral testosterone can also harm the liver, and this side effect is most likely the sole reason behind the Chapter 1 myth that testosterone causes liver damage. High doses of oral, synthetic androgens are absorbed into the entero-hepatic circu-lation and may adversely affect the liver, while subcutaneous pellets and topical patches avoid the entero-hepatic circulation and bypass the liver. Oral testosterone may also increase the risk of deep venous thrombosis or pulmonary embolism. With oral testosterone, there are more gallbladder problems, and you have to take those pills every day, so your hormone levels are going up and down like a roller-coaster. There are clearly more GI upset and nausea, and you're not going to get the same constant blood levels that you can get with other hormones.

Sublingual/Buccal

Sublingual and buccal testosterone delivery work by either placing a dissolving tablet under the tongue (sublingual) or by placing a tablet against the surface of the gums (buccal). It is different from oral delivery in that very little of the substance is swallowed, avoiding potential liver toxicity.

Transdermal

Transdermal refers to topical delivery through the skin by the use of a patch, gel, or cream. Transdermal testosterone is usually applied to the skin twice daily. To efficiently deliver testosterone into the body, chemical enhancers are added to the patch to increase permeability of the skin, and these enhancers often cause irritation and/or allergic reactions. When you use patches, the absorption can be poor; in fact, sometimes 45 percent of people do not absorb the hormones from their patch. In addition, you have to put them on daily or twice a day. Since blood levels vary from person to person, the levels of testosterone achieved in some women utilizing creams parallel those of their male partners. Yikes! Too much testosterone is not optimal and can cause increased side effects. It's very difficult to get unique optimal blood levels, and the rollercoaster ride of blood levels often results in women stopping their testosterone therapy. In addition, you can transfer those hormones to other people, children, and pets.

Injectable

Injectable synthetic testosterone in women causes very high serum levels and a plethora of androgen-related side effects. There's pain at the injection site because all of the injectables are in an oil base. There are also allergies to the cottonseed oil, and there are more erythrocytosis, more red blood cell mass, and more aromatization, meaning more of the testosterone gets converted to estrogen because of the high blood levels. The increase in estradiol levels contributes to additional breast tenderness, weight gain, and swelling. Rarely are testosterone injections an acceptable choice to optimize testosterone in women.

Pellets

Pellets provide a more consistent blood level over time because the testosterone is released slowly over a period of weeks or months. A pellet composed of bioidentical testosterone is implanted beneath the skin. The pellets are about the size of a grain of rice and are typically placed in the buttocks or abdomen. The insertion of the pellet is a quick procedure, usually done under local anesthesia. Pellets are typically replaced after three to four months. The advantages of pellets are that hormone optimization and consistent blood levels are easily achievable. You don't have the rollercoaster effect. Pellets are available in many doses, allowing for individualization of therapy. Insertion is usually painless, performed under local anesthesia, and you can quickly return to normal activities. Although pellets occasionally work their way out through the incision, the incidence of extrusions in females is less than 1 percent.

11

COMPOUNDING—THE PERSONALIZED APPROACH TO PRECISION MEDICINE AND GENESIS FOR TESTOSTERONE HORMONE OPTIMIZATION

As you've discovered in previous chapters, testosterone therapy for women actually antedates testosterone therapy for men. In the first five years after its initial synthesis, testosterone was tried in a number of clinical situations with success. In fact, it was prescribed to treat the symptoms of surgical menopause in women as early as 1936. Testosterone therapy for the treatment of women with normally occurring menopause dates back to 1939, when it was utilized for the treatment of postmenopausal osteoporosis.

Clearly, testosterone for women is not new! Since 2004, study after study has confirmed that testosterone is breast-protective, heart-protective, bone-protective, and brain-protective for women. It is even included in WHO's 2019 Twenty-first Edition List of Essential Medicines—the safest and most effective medicines needed in a health system. Yet even to this day, there is no FDA-approved product for women, which also means there is no Big Pharma product or solution.

However, do not get mad that your most important hormone has been overlooked by the pharmaceutical industry and the FDA. The absence of FDA approval may be a blessing in disguise.

What is the difference between pharmaceutical compounding and pharmaceutical manufacturing?

There are two types of medications that can be prescribed for you. One is a compounded medication, and the other is a Big Pharma medication. (There are also over-the-counter [OTC] medications, but they do not require a prescription.)

Pharmaceutical compounding is the science responsible for the creation of personalized medicine. Compounding combines individual ingredients in the exact strength and dosage form required by the patient to better support his or her own unique needs. Compounded medications are ordered by a licensed physician or other prescriber and must be mixed in a safe and carefully controlled environment by a licensed compounding pharmacist. Compounding allows for the appropriately prescribed treatment to be completely customized based on the patient's hormone levels, symptoms, and health concerns. Just as aging is a unique process, hormone optimization for women requires a unique individualized therapy.

Pharmaceutical manufacturing (Big Pharma) is the process used to formulate and create commercially available drugs. Unlike compounding, Big Pharma (Merck & Co., Pfizer, Johnson & Johnson, etc.) creates drugs in preset formulas or doses on an industrial scale. Big Pharma manufactures millions of doses or formulas every year. The dose in each pill, capsule, and so forth is the same no matter who is taking it; the drug dosage is typically based on the patient's weight. Instead of one pill, an individual may take two, or a pill can be cut in half or crushed, but that can result in deviations from the recommended dosage (and the difference between a therapeutic dose and one that is toxic or ineffective is sometimes a very narrow margin).

Big Pharma would like you to believe that its drugs are superior—and safer—solutions, but the reality is very different. Studies have shown that most drugs prescribed in the United States are effective in fewer than 60 percent of treated patients. For example, at least 70 percent of patients who take the cardiovascular drugs known as ACE inhibitors and beta-blockers, nearly 40 percent of the people prescribed antidepressants, and at least 30 percent of both the patients given statins for high cholesterol and those given beta2-agonists for asthma realize little or no benefit.

According to a 2014 report from the Edmond J. Safra Center for Ethics at Harvard University, new prescription drugs have a one-in-five chance of causing serious reactions after they have been approved. A review of hospital charts revealed that even properly prescribed drugs cause about 1.9 million hospitalizations a year, and another 840,000 hospitalized patients are given drugs that cause serious adverse reactions for a total of 2.74 million serious adverse drug reactions. About 128,000 people die from drugs prescribed to them, making prescription drugs a major health risk, ranking fourth with stroke as a leading cause of death.

Unlike Big Pharma, which originated in the second half of the 19th century, compounding is not new. Between 130 and 200 AD, Galen of Pergamon, a Greek physician, surgeon, and philosopher in the Roman Empire, introduced compounding and the process of mixing two or more medicines to meet the individual needs of a patient.

A compounded medication seems like a superior solution. After all, you, your body, and your health issues are unique. They're not the same as those of your next-door neighbor. So why did the medical world move from compounding for one specific patient to Big Pharma? It had to do with profit and economies of scale and not lack of skills or knowledge.

This is a very important piece of information to keep in mind: the primary reason Big Pharma exists is not because there was anything wrong with compounding but because it was just not scalable. So once it became about the economies of scalability, Big Pharma had to figure out a way to standardize the amount that existed in each one of the batches and then make it available to millions of people.

Now, it's great that antibiotics, antipyretics, and all these mass-produced medications that we're giving people are pharmaceutically made, but compounding is the only way to give the individual patient what they specifically need.

Compounding Today: A Superior, Personalized Solution and the Cornerstone of Precision Medicine

So what does compounding look like this decade? Interestingly enough, it's everywhere around you. When most people think of a compounded medication, they assume it's a capsule, cream, or gel. But compounded medications are also created as a liquid to be swallowed or injected. All the IV meds with the vitamins in them administered in a hospital, clinic, or office are considered compounded products. Chemotherapy is compounded. If a medication arrives in a powder form and needs to be reconstituted, effectively changing its form, it has been compounded. Last but not least, there are hormones.

The American College of Obstetricians and Gynecologists (ACOG), the North American Menopause Society, and the Endocrine Society have all yet to figure out the value of testosterone for women beyond as a therapy for hypoactive sexual dysphoric disorder. They have all overlooked the fact that testosterone therapy has been used for eighty years in five continents for the symptoms of pre- and post-menopause. Think about all those symptoms that their patients have in every category; subcutaneous compounded testosterone pellet therapy improves those symptoms and improves quality of life.

There is no FDA-approved testosterone preparation for the treatment of testosterone insufficiency in women. However, for the past eighty years, androgen replacement has been used off-label to treat testosterone deficiency or insufficiency in women. There really is no basis for most of the reference ranges; in fact, the literature as reported by the Princeton Consensus Group declared there are no normal testosterone levels in women. What you see on the lab slip are expected levels, which are levels that could occur in any woman from age twenty to eighty.

Furthermore, serum levels haven't been found even to correlate with the presence or absence of symptoms. Normal levels don't mean testosterone replacement will not be effective, and so many women who've had their levels tested and who have symptoms have been told, "You don't need testosterone; you don't need hormones," even though they would have benefited. Instead, they were placed on multiple Big Pharma medications to treat the symptoms rather than find and treat the root cause. If a normal testosterone level is found, it should not be used to rule out a deficiency in women or become the sole determining factor in making that decision to treat testosterone insufficiency as a clinical syndrome.

We've got to treat the patient, not the lab. For so long, everybody has wanted to define testosterone insufficiency or deficiency with a lab value. That just doesn't occur. It's a clinical syndrome. It doesn't occur at any definitive threshold. I can't tell you at what number or value a patient will start having symptoms, but what I can tell you is the symptoms of testosterone deficiency are clear, and treating those symptoms is easy. Treating those symptoms, not the lab, is what improves people's quality of life.

With compounding, we can individualize hormone optimization for everyone. And here's a surprising (big deal) benefit for patients when their healthcare is personalized and their hormones are optimized as follows.

One of my patients drove from her home in Del Rio, Texas, to my Houston office to see me, and she said, "Oh, my God. You've helped me so much. I feel so much better." I said, "Yeah. By the way, did you recognize that your diabetes is gone?" She said, "Yeah, that's great, but that's not the big deal. The big deal is every morning I get up, I feel pretty. I never felt pretty in my whole life." Testosterone mattered . . . more—again! Another life changed!

Look, the industry needs to stop harming people. Quit putting Band-Aids on people. Just keep it simple. Keep your solutions personalized. That's what I do at BioTE® Medical, LLC. Remember: changing lives is fascinating. Together, if we change enough lives, we can change healthcare.

12

LET'S END THE DEBATE: TESTOSTERONE MATTERS . . . MORE!

As we were going to press with *Testosterone Matters . . . More!*, the *Journal of American Medical Association* (*JAMA*) published an article entitled "Which Postmenopausal Women Should Use Testosterone for Low Sexual Desire?" The article begins, "Sarah uses kitchen measuring spoons to dispense just the right dose—between a pinch and a smidge—of testosterone gel formulated for men to treat her low sexual desire."

A pinch? A smidge? Solely to treat low sexual desire? That single sentence from an article published in 2020 in the prestigious *JAMA* sums up the cavalier attitude many in the medical community have towards women's health.

If this book accomplishes one thing, I hope it's that you and all our medical colleagues understand women's health is not just about sex drive.

As many of you have discovered, there is a clinical need to have some form of HRT. As a result, serious practitioners have turned to bioidentical hormone replacement therapy (BHRT) and experienced overwhelmingly positive results.

Figure 8: Androgens peak in women in their twenties.

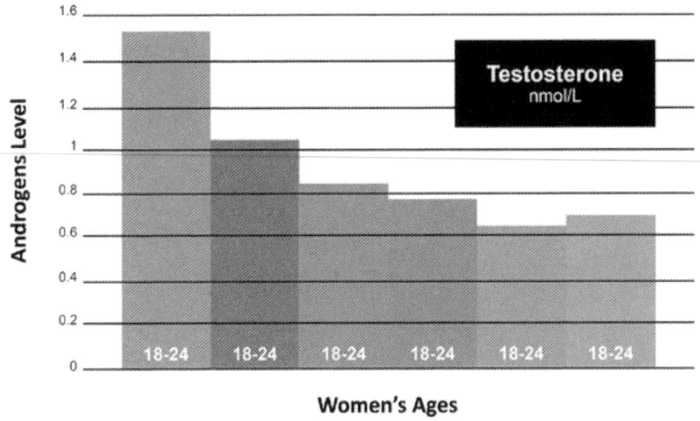

Low testosterone in women creates an increased risk of:

- Alzheimer's disease
- cardiovascular disease
- osteoporotic-related fractures
- diabetes mellitus
- possibly cancer

While there is no FDA-approved testosterone preparation for the treatment of testosterone insufficiency in women, most commercial assays for the measurement of free testosterone and total testosterone are based on male data. The lack of sensitivity and precision required to measure these very low levels makes it difficult, even using liquid chromatography.

We've got to treat the patient, not the lab.

Hormones are idiosyncratic. Therefore, HRT is a personalized therapy that requires practitioners to individually evaluate each patient, make case-by-case clinical determinations, and provide unique, customized treatments.

This is why bioidentical hormones and compounding are both so integral to HRT.

Physiological data and clinical outcomes demonstrate that bioidentical hormones are associated with lower risks (including the risk of breast cancer and CVD) and are more efficacious than their synthetic and animal-derived counterparts.

Because bioidentical hormones are structurally identical to endogenous hormones, they are able to bond with human hormone receptors in the exact same manner as endogenous hormones. Synthetic hormones, by contrast, are dissimilar to endogenous hormones except for the portion of their chemical structure that binds to the human body's receptors.

Because synthetic hormones have a different chemical structure, the synthetic hormone molecule may bind to the human hormone receptors in one tissue but not in others, and it might bind to other receptors that the endogenous hormone will not.

The failure of synthetic hormones to bind with all of the same receptors as endogenous hormones, as well as their binding to other non-endogenous hormone receptors, creates adverse effects (e.g., tumors).

- Given the preventative nature of HRT and the lack of a standardized patient condition that requires HRT, compounded products are the natural fit.

- Bioidentical hormone replacement therapy (BHRT) is personalized medicine, and such compounded medications provide practitioners with the flexibility necessary to provide treatment that, in their clinical opinions, is optimal for the health of each of their patients.

- Compounding allows us to accurately dose patients, customize medication based on patients' individual specific needs, use medications with higher quality standards than are offered by (or required of) commercial manufacturers (e.g., lower-potency variations), and give patients significantly greater access to medications required by their therapies.

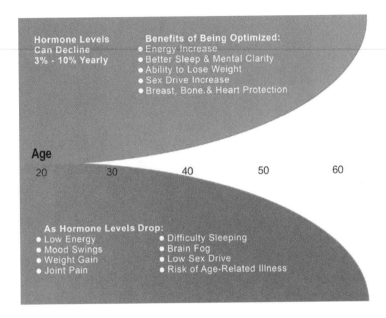

Hormone Levels Can Decline 3% - 10% Yearly

Benefits of Being Optimized:
- Energy Increase
- Better Sleep & Mental Clarity
- Ability to Lose Weight
- Sex Drive Increase
- Breast, Bone, & Heart Protection

Age
20   30   40   50   60

As Hormone Levels Drop:
- Low Energy
- Mood Swings
- Weight Gain
- Joint Pain
- Difficulty Sleeping
- Brain Fog
- Low Sex Drive
- Risk of Age-Related Illness

Since 2006, I have performed over sixty-six thousand subcutaneous bioidentical hormone pellet procedures on more than twenty thousand patients with less than 1 percent experiencing complications. Ninety-five percent of my patients have their hormones optimized after their first round of therapy.

My patients include:

- Premenopausal women with testosterone insufficiency
- Menopausal women with testosterone insufficiency
- Breast cancer survivors
- Patients whose symptoms were not effectively treated with commercially available products
- Patients seeking to reduce their risks of disease, most notably CVD

Figure 8

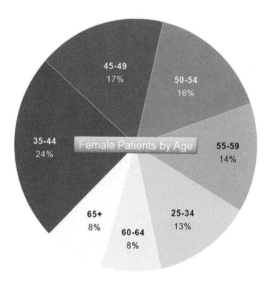

My hope is that *Testosterone Matters . . . More!* has helped illuminate the importance of treating the patient, not the lab, and has shown the benefits of testosterone in BHRT.

Safe and Effective. Research and clinical experience show that bioidentical hormones are safe and effective and the adverse effects that have been seen in the past from HRT stem from the use of synthetic hormones.

Compounds Are Necessary. Hormones are inherently idiosyncratic, which means BHRT is a form of personalized medicine that requires practitioners to individually evaluate each case. As such, practitioners need the flexibility that compounded (as opposed to commercial) bioidentical hormone products can offer.

Practitioner Discretion and Education. Because of the idiosyncratic nature of hormones, patients necessarily rely upon the judgment and analysis of practitioners. We need to continue to empower practitioners to work with their patients to proactively address their individual healthcare needs and desires, and part of that process includes educating practitioners on BHRT.

Highest Quality. Bioidentical hormone replacement therapy is making its way to the forefront of medicine as it gets adopted by an increasing number of practitioners who come from a wide array of specialties. We BHRT practitioners want to make sure that the compounded products we use are made pursuant to the heightened specifications we require and are of the highest quality.

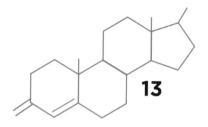

13

TESTOSTERONE MATTERS . . . MORE— FOR YOUR MALE PARTNER TOO!

After reading this book, you may begin noticing that your husband, partner, or significant other is displaying similar symptoms to yours: he's grumpy, tired, unenthusiastic, and uninterested in doing many of the things you and he once enjoyed. He's even starting to become a bit forgetful and less interested in intimate relations with you.

He may have low testosterone.

CASE HISTORY FROM A PRACTITIONER
Judson Brandeis, MD, Board-Certified Urologist and Expert in the Field of Men's Health

Christopher's Story

I could tell from the way that Christopher walked through the front door that the past few years had been rough. It was obvious from the way that he carried himself that at one time he had been an athlete, but now he was overweight and out of shape. His hairline was receding dramatically, and his forehead wrinkles were deep ravines.

When we finally sat down to talk, Christopher looked

older than his stated age of fifty-nine. He confided in me that his marriage of twenty-three years was on the rocks and that he had not been physically intimate with his wife in three years. Viagra used to work for him, but now it was inconsistent, and he was scared to try and fail again. He thought that once his kids left the house, things would get better, but his wife just did not seem interested anymore.

In order to compensate, he threw himself back into work. However, it seemed that time had passed him by. He was no match for the millennials, with their iPhones and Google docs and apps for seemingly every task. Ten years ago, his sales numbers were tops in the company, and he even won a trip to Hawaii with the corporate leadership team. Now a big trip was to the grocery store. Unfortunately, these days he was buying more alcohol and too much comfort food. His most exciting recent purchase was an eighty-inch flat-screen television, and by now he had worn a hole in his favorite couch pillow.

It was difficult for Christopher to sleep because his financial worries were keeping him up. He was still making decent money, but two college tuitions were draining the family savings. He had always promised his children that they would leave college without debt. However, he had not anticipated how expensive college was going to be.

When Christopher came back with his labs, the results were not unexpected. His testosterone was 289 with a free testosterone of 6.3; both levels were at the very low end. His cholesterol level was abnormally high at 273 with high triglycerides, and his sugar levels showed prediabetes.

As a board-certified urologist and male rejuvenation specialist, I sat down with Christopher, and we had a difficult discussion about his downward life spiral. His situation is typical for the men that I see: men who at one time were on top of the world—raising families, supporting communities, building careers—but the vitality of youth had left them, and they were not prepared for what came next.

Christopher and I put together a treatment plan that included testosterone supplementation using the BioTE method of hormone optimization, nitric-oxide boosting with AFFIRM, tadalafil 5mg daily dose, and shockwave therapy.

The placement of the testosterone pellets took five minutes, and Christopher was on his way. I saw him once a week for the next twelve weeks when he came in for his shockwave therapy. By the second week, it was clear that something was different about Christopher. His mood was improving. He said that his wife and daughter have clearly seen a difference in his outlook and attitude. When he came in for his third shockwave treatment, Christopher told us that he had joined a gym and had started working out with a personal trainer.

By the fifth week, Christopher came in looking less fatigued. His testosterone levels came back at 1296 with a free testosterone of 22.3. His hematocrit was 48.6, which is within the normal range. When my nurse inquired, Christopher noted that he had been sleeping a lot better. He confided in us that his coworkers have been impressed with his energy level and attention to detail and that his sales numbers had improved.

The following week, Christopher was blushing. With a slight smile, he motioned to me to come into his treatment room and close the door. He confided that he had been physically intimate with his wife for the first time in nearly three years. Tears welled up in his eyes as he spoke about how difficult the lack of physical intimacy had been on his marriage. He said that he was constantly worried that his wife was looking at other men because of his impotence. For the first time in many years, he was hopeful about his marriage.

Christopher clearly had made a commitment to his personal wellness. Since his testosterone was at excellent levels, he was able to build muscle and get rid of some of his excess fat. His posture was clearly improved. I could hear Christopher bragging to my nurses that he had lost twenty pounds and he was not going to stop there. After twelve weeks, Christopher had completed his course of shockwave therapy. His erectile function had significantly improved, as well as his overall outlook on life.

Two months later and five months after his initial pellet implantation, I saw that Christopher was on the schedule for a follow-up pellet implantation. When he walked into the office, I hardly recognized him. He had managed to keep the weight off and build some muscle. His eyes were full of energy and positivity. Even his new clothes seemed to fit better. He confided in me that his relationship with his wife had never been better and that after the shock-wave therapy, he no longer needed to use Cialis. That was two years ago, and Christopher has brought his wife in for testosterone supplementation, as well as half of his men's softball team.

In our late teens and twenties, male testosterone levels are around 900 or higher. We feel the vitality of youth and build muscle and careers. Over time, testosterone slowly declines. In men, testosterone levels decline 1 to 1.5 percent per year after age thirty, and the "Hypogonadism in Males" study estimates the prevalence of low testosterone (total testosterone less than 300 nanograms/deciliter) is as high as 38.7 percent in males over forty-five. After age thirty-five, testosterone levels may decline 20 percent per decade. The aging process is candles on a birthday cake, but also certain physiologic processes like testosterone production predictably decline. Not everyone declines at the same rate or to the same level, but, over time, everybody's levels decrease. The problem is that testosterone deficiency in men, as in women, is a clinical syndrome. There are many more men suffering from testosterone deficiency who may not have laboratory values less than 300 nanograms per deciliter.

Men with suspicious signs or symptoms of androgen deficiency, or low testosterone, need confirmatory biochemical testing before the diagnosis is made. It is not known the exact biochemical threshold of serum testosterone concentration below which symptoms of androgen deficiency and adverse outcomes occur. Signs of low testosterone include a decrease in libido, lack of energy, decrease in strength, loss of height, decreased enjoyment of life, sadness, sexual problems, reduced athletic performance, fatigue, and reduced work performance. Other issues include a general decline in physical and mental well-being, sweating, sleep problems, irritability, nervousness, anxiety, a decrease in morning erections, and a feeling of being burnt out.

One of the earliest signs of low testosterone is a decline in libido or sex drive. There are so many factors in life that can influence libido that your partner may not notice that it has declined.

Job stress, marital stress, parenting stress, and other normal aspects of life that increase stress hormones can have a negative effect on libido. By the time your partner realizes it, your romantic relationship has evaporated. Testosterone also affects the inner lining of the penis. Without testosterone, the lining of the erectile bodies becomes shrunken and stiff.

Signs of low testosterone include:

1. Decrease in libido
2. Penile shrinkage
3. Memory, focus, and concentration issues
4. Sarcopenia or muscle loss
5. Loss of bone mineral density
6. Insulin resistance increasing risk of diabetes
7. Increase risk of heart disease, high blood pressure, and abnormal lipid profile, also known as metabolic syndrome
8. Insomnia
9. Joint pain

What is a normal testosterone level? Normal levels range between 300 and 1,000. Unfortunately, other factors influence how the body responds to this important hormone. A man's receptors may be damaged from toxins as he ages, he may not have enough vitamins and other cellular cofactors for his cells to be able to utilize the testosterone in his bloodstream, and his cells may suffer from senility and function at attenuated levels. However, the need to replace testosterone depends on symptoms rather than a lab test.

How is testosterone made? The testicles have cells called Leydig cells that make testosterone. Ninety percent of the mass of the testicle is used to make sperm, and 10 percent is used to make testosterone. Testosterone is delivered into the vascular system. The Leydig cells are regulated by signals from the pituitary gland, which is at the base of the brain. The pituitary gland releases luteinizing hormone (LH), which stimulates the Leydig cells to make testosterone.

Testosterone undergoes a chemical reaction in fat cells that turns some of the testosterone into estrogen. This is called aromatization. We think of testosterone and estrogen as very different molecules, but in actuality the difference between the testosterone and the estrogen molecules is one hydrogen molecule. Hydrogen is the smallest unit of matter. Increasing estrogens shut down the pituitary gland, which will then shut down the production of LH, which causes the testosterone level to decline. Over half of obese men have low testosterone. Diabetes also increases the risk of low testosterone. If a man has diabetes, he has a 50 percent chance of having low testosterone. If he has diabetes and is obese, the chances of having low testosterone are greater than 80 percent.

Excessive alcohol use can cause liver damage, which increases the production of sex-hormone-binding globulin (SHBG), which is a protein that binds to testosterone and prevents it from binding to the testosterone receptor.

When taking testosterone exogenously, meaning through shots, creams, or pellets, testicles produce less testosterone. The outside testosterone circulates to the pituitary gland, where it signals the pituitary gland to stop making testosterone. The pituitary also stops making follicle-stimulating hormone (FHS). Since 90 percent of the mass of the testicle is used to make sperm, the testicle begins to shrink. It is not unusual to experience a 10 to 15 percent reduction in the size of the testicles from testosterone therapy.

Side effects of testosterone replacement therapy include some mild and temporary leg swelling. If a man has high levels of testosterone, he may develop acne or some nipple tenderness. Testosterone can also overstimulate red blood cell production, which will increase hematocrit, which is another name for blood count.

If his blood count gets too high, his physician may request that he donate blood to bring it back to the normal range. Testosterone can also aggravate sleep apnea in about one-third of men who have this disorder.

Prostate cancer is one of the most common cancers in men, but it is not more common in men on testosterone replacement. In fact, studies have shown that low testosterone levels in men increase their risk of prostate cancer and for a more aggressive tumor(s) should they develop the disease. Low serum testosterone levels are predictive of prostate cancer. It is important to get his PSA monitored once a year while he is on testosterone replacement therapy. Replacing testosterone in a man who has been successfully treated for prostate cancer has been shown to be safe.

Serum testosterone levels peak in the morning and decline over the course of the day as a result of circadian rhythms. Most normal ranges for testosterone levels are established using a morning blood sample. The effect of circadian rhythm is blunted with aging. There are day-to-day intraindividual variations in the level of testosterone.

Serum total testosterone concentration represents both protein-bound and unbound testosterone in circulation. Bioavailable testosterone refers to unbound testosterone and albumin-bound testosterone that is relatively disassociated. Free or bioavailable testosterone concentration should be measured when total testosterone levels are at the lower limit of the normal range or when altered SHBG levels are suspected.

Randomized controlled studies have shown that testosterone therapy provides several positive improvements in body composition, metabolic control, and psychological and sexual parameters.

Erectile dysfunction (ED), along with sexual dysfunction, is the most specific predictor of androgen deficiency. When an erection is restored by PDE 5 inhibitors (Cialis or Viagra), the addition of testosterone therapy does not result in further benefit of erectile function. For ED refractory to PDE 5 inhibitors, testosterone therapy has the potential to improve ED and lower the dependence on PDE 5 inhibitors.

Increased awareness has been given to the interplay between testosterone and various aspects of cardiovascular health. In addition, and of great concern, low testosterone levels are associated with increased mortality as was shown in Shore's study in 2006. Shore's study results were reinforced by Khaw's study in 2007, wherein 11,606 men aged forty to seventy-nine years participated and were surveyed from 1993 to 1997 and then followed up to 2003. Khaw concluded that low testosterone levels were associated with significantly greater all-cause mortality, cardiovascular mortality, and cancer mortality.

A study published in 2016 by Sharma et al. examined 83,010 male veterans with documented low testosterone levels. Optimizing their testosterone levels was associated with a significant reduction in all-cause mortality, myocardial infarction, and stroke. A second study by Sharma published in 2017 concluded that testosterone optimization is associated with a significant decrease in the incidence of atrial fibrillation (the most common cardiac dysrhythmia associated with significant morbidity and mortality). Moreover, a negative correlation has been demonstrated among endogenous testosterone and severity of coronary artery disease, congestive heart failure, and thickness of the walls of blood vessels.

Despite all the studies, there has been a considerable degree of misinformation and confusion regarding testosterone treatment, due in large part to two reports suggesting increased cardiovascular risk: one published in November 2013 by Vigen et al. and one published in January 2014 by Finkle et al. Two days later, the US FDA announced it would investigate cardiovascular risk with testosterone products. The media fed the fires of confusion with articles and opinion pieces on the dangers of testosterone therapy on the basis of these two reports, and it will come as no surprise that much of the information regarding indications, benefits, and risk of testosterone therapy was erroneous or distorted. Since 2014, there have been numerous reports and studies in excellent peer-reviewed journals that have conclusively demonstrated the benefits of testosterone optimization on cardiovascular health.

Maintaining normal testosterone levels plays an important role in cardiovascular health. Optimizing men's testosterone levels with androgen deficiency improves myocardial ischemia, exercise capability, and cardiovascular risk factors. However, current available guidelines do not recommend offering androgen-deprivation screening to patients with heart disease, nor do they recommend supplementing testosterone therapy to improve cardiovascular outcomes. It is interesting that practitioners treat men with statins that increase their risk of fatigue, cognitive decline, diabetes, and ED; however, only 1 to 2 percent of males benefit from a reduction in cardiovascular events. On the other hand, testosterone optimization improves blood flow to the heart, reduces visceral fat, improves insulin resistance, and reduces plaque formation in the coronaries. That is why testosterone matters . . . more in men too!

As you can see, low testosterone in men is not just about erections, just as low testosterone in women is not just about libido. It affects the health of every major system in the body. Once a man's testosterone is optimized, his whole quality of life and overall well-being are better: total cholesterol and triglycerides are decreased, HDL (good cholesterol) is increased, lean body mass is significantly increased, anxiety and irritability are decreased, and cognitive clarity is improved. If testosterone deficiency is not treated and not optimized, men are in danger of developing the same health risks that we've explored in this book: an increase in Alzheimer's, CVD, osteoporotic fractures, prostate cancer and the severity of prostate cancer, diabetes, and sarcopenia or muscle loss.

If your partner seems like the poster model for testosterone deficiency, I am including the health assessment for men (male symptom questionnaire: Figure 9) for you to go over with him. It will certainly help him see if he is a candidate for testosterone therapy.

Figure 9

bioTE MEDICAL

Health Assessment For Men (Male Symptom Questionnaire)

Name: _____ Date: _____

E-Mail Address: _____

Which of the following symptoms apply to you currently (in the last 2 weeks)? Please mark the appropriate box for each symptom. For symptoms that do not currently apply or no longer apply, mark "never".

Symptoms	Never (0)	Mild (1)	Moderate (2)	Severe (3)	Very Severe (4)
Sweating (night sweats or excessive sweating)					
Sleep problems (difficulty falling asleep, sleeping through the night or waking up too early)					
Increased need for sleep or falls asleep easily after a meal					
Depressive mood (feeling down, sad, lack of drive)					
Irritability (mood swings, feeling aggressive, angers easily)					
Anxiety (inner restlessness, feeling panicky, feeling nervous, inner tension)					
Physical exhaustion (general decrease in muscle strength or endurance, decrease in work performance, fatigue, lack of energy, stamina or motivation)					
Sexual problems (change in sexual desire or in sexual performance)					
Bladder problems (difficulty in urinating, increased need to urinate)					
Erectile changes (less strong erections, loss of morning erections)					
Joint and muscular symptoms (joint pain or swelling, muscle weakness, poor recovery after exercise)					
Difficulties with memory					
Problems with thinking, concentrating or reasoning					
Difficulty learning new things					
Trouble thinking of the right word to describe persons, places or things when speaking					
Increase in frequency or intensity of headaches/migraines					
Rapid hair loss or thinning					
Feel cold all the time or have cold hands or feet					
Weight gain, increased belly fat, or difficulty losing weight despite diet and exercise					
Infrequent or absent ejaculations					
Total:					

Severity	Score
Mild	1 - 20
Moderate	21 - 40
Severe	41 - 60
Very Severe	61 - 80

Male Health Assessment   Revision Date: 01_27_20

In October 2015, an international expert consensus conference regarding testosterone deficiency and its treatment was held in Prague, Czech Republic. The meeting was sponsored by King's College London and the International Society for the Study of the Aging Male, and it was held in response to all the misinformation and confusion in the medical community. Nine statements, termed "resolutions," were discussed by participants (representing a broad range of specialties from eleven countries on four continents). All nine resolutions received unanimous approval.

Figure 10

MAYO CLINIC PROCEEDINGS

TABLE 1. Resolutions of the International Expert Consensus Conference on Testosterone Deficiency and Its Treatment

Resolutions	Expert comments
1. TD is a well-established, significant medical condition that negatively affects male sexuality, reproduction, general health, and quality of life	○ TD (low levels of testosterone) • May predict increased risk of developing diabetes, metabolic syndrome • Contributes to decreased bone mineral density • Is associated with increased all-cause and cardiovascular mortality • Negatively impacts general health and quality of life
2. The symptoms and signs of TD occur as a result of low levels of T and may benefit from treatment regardless of whether there is an identified underlying etiology	• Symptoms and signs of TD occur in healthy volunteers or patients who undergo androgen deprivation; these symptoms and signs resolve with T normalization • Historically recognized causes of TD are rare (eg, anorchia, craniopharyngioma, pituitary tumor), recently termed *classical* hypogonadism. These conditions account for only a tiny fraction of men with TD • TD occurs frequently with conditions other than "classical" causes • No evidence exists to support restriction of T therapy only to men with known underlying etiology
3. TD is a global public health concern	• Prevalence rates in men range from 2% to 38% in studies from Asia, Europe, North America, and South America • Variation in prevalence rates can be explained by differences in the operative definition of TD and biochemical thresholds • A US study estimates an additional $190-$525 billion in health care expenditures over 20 years due to TD
4. T therapy for men with TD is effective, rational, and evidence based	○ High-level evidence shows T therapy effectively: • Increases sexual desire (libido) and erectile and orgasmic function • Increases lean body mass • Decreases fat mass • Improves bone mineral density ○ Strongly suggestive evidence for improvement in mood, energy
5. There is no T concentration threshold that reliably distinguishes those who will respond to treatment from those who will not	No study has revealed a single testosterone threshold that reliably separates those who experience signs and symptoms of TD from those who do not, nor who will likely respond to treatment. Interpretation of total T concentrations is confounded by: • Interindividual variation • Variation in serum SHBG (binds tightly to T, removing it from the bioavailable pool) • Genetic variation in androgen sensitivity due to AR gene polymorphisms (number of CAG repeats) Free T can be a useful indicator of androgen status
6. There is no scientific basis for any age-specific recommendations against the use of T therapy in men	• The term *age-related hypogonadism* is of questionable validity since the decline in mean serum T level with age is minor and primarily attributable to comorbidities, especially obesity • Older men respond well to T therapy, as do younger men • Increased risk of erythrocytosis in older men requires monitoring but does not merit withholding T therapy if indicated • It is illogical to single out TD as the one medical condition among many (eg, diabetes, hypertension, heart disease, cancer, arthritis) that does not merit treatment because it becomes more prevalent with age

Continued on next page

TABLE 1. Continued	
Resolutions	Expert comments
7. The evidence does not support increased risks of CV events with T therapy	• Two observational studies received intense media attention after reporting increased CV risks. Both had major flaws/limitations. One misreported results, the other had no control group • Low serum T is associated with increased atherosclerosis, coronary artery disease, obesity, diabetes, and mortality • Several RCTs in men with known heart disease (angina, heart failure) showed greater benefits with T vs placebo (greater time to ischemia, greater exercise capacity) • The largest meta-analysis showed no increased risk with T therapy; reduced risk was noted in men with metabolic conditions • No increased risk of venothrombotic events with T therapy
8. The evidence does not support increased risk of PCa with T therapy	• Serum androgen concentrations are not associated with increased risk of PCa nor aggressive disease • T therapy has no greater risk of PCa than placebo • Aggressive/high-grade PCa is associated with low serum T levels • Early data suggest no increased risk of recurrence/progression with T therapy in men previously treated for PCa
9. The evidence supports a major research initiative to explore possible benefits of T therapy for cardiometabolic disease, including diabetes	• A large body of evidence suggests lower serum T concentrations are associated with increased CV risk; higher levels are protective • T therapy reliably increases lean mass, decreases fat mass, and may improve glycemic control • Mortality rates are reduced by half in men with TD who received T therapy compared with untreated men in observational studies • Among men who received T therapy, those with normalized T levels had a reduced rate of CV events/mortality vs men with persistently low T

CAG = cytosine, adenine, guanine; CV = cardiovascular; PCa = prostate cancer; RCT = randomized controlled trial; SHBG = sex hormone–binding globulin; T = testosterone; TD = testosterone deficiency.

Mayo Clin Proc., July 2016: 91(7):881-896, http://dx.doi.org/10.1016/j.mayocp.2016.04.007
www.mayoclinicproceedings.org

Clearly, testosterone for men deserves its own book!

If your husband, partner, or significant other is experiencing the symptoms in the assessment, please consider sharing this book and especially this chapter with him. Testosterone optimization will help both of you feel better, age healthier, and live happier.

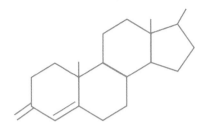

ABOUT THE AUTHOR
GARY S. DONOVITZ, MD, FACOG

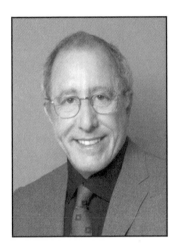

Gary Donovitz, MD, FACOG, is leading a healthcare revolution that focuses on optimizing and balancing bioidentical hormones for aging healthier and living happier by supporting heart, bone, brain, and sexual health, improved energy and clarity, and happiness for men and women of all ages.

After practicing as a board-certified OB/GYN for thirty years, Dr. Donovitz is now an internationally recognized leader, speaker, educator, and advocate of hormone optimization. He is the founder and chairman of BioTE® Medical, LLC, a leading innovator in subcutaneous hormone pellet therapy. He has personally performed more than fifty thousand pellet insertions. The BioTE state-of-the-art training facility hosts physicians, healthcare providers, and medical staff members monthly during the BioTE Method learning and certification process. Over four thousand practitioners in more than two thousand clinics nationwide have successfully completed his rigorous curriculum and clinical training program, ensuring the highest safety, efficacy, and results for every patient. Collectively, these practitioners have performed more than 1.7 million pellet insertions to date.

His commitment to constantly raise the bar for healthcare extends beyond hormone therapy, as Dr. Donovitz has been at the forefront of developments in robotic surgery and has trained physicians across the country on how to perform operations using these advances in technology.

Dr. Donovitz received the Isadore Dyer Award for best teaching resident while studying at Tulane University in New Orleans, Louisiana. He is a fellow of the American College of Obstetrics and Gynecology, a fellow of the Royal Society of Medicine, chairman of the International Consensus Committee on Testosterone Use in Women, and founder of the Institute for Hormonal Balance.

After monitoring outcomes for over 850,000 men and women who have benefited from BioTE hormone optimization, results continue to exceed expectations with more than 96 percent of patients satisfied.

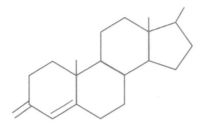

RESOURCES

Chapter One

Dimitrakakis, C., R. Glaser, and A. York. "Beneficial effects of testosterone therapy in women measured by the validated Menopause Rating Scale (MRS)." *Maturitas* 68, no. 4 (2011): 355–361.

Glaser, R. "Testosterone therapy in women: Myths and misconceptions." *Maturitas* 74, no. 3 (2013): 230–34.

Glaser, R., et al. "Testosterone implants in women: Pharmacologic doses for a physiologic effect." *Maturitas* 74, no. 3 (2013): 179–184.

Glaser, R., A. York, and C. Dimitrakakis. "Effect of testosterone therapy on the female voice." *Climacteric* 19, no. 2 (2016): 198–203. https://doi.org/10.3109/13697137.2015.1136925.

Glaser, R. L., C. Dimitrakakis, and A. G. Messenger. "Improvement in scalp hair growth in androgen-deficient women treated with testosterone: a questionnaire study." *British Journal of Dermatology* 166, no. 2 (2012): 274–278. https://doi.org/10.111 1/j.1365-2133.2011.10655.

Donovitz, Gary, MD, et al. "Testosterone Insufficiency and Treatment in Women: International Expert Consensus." *Medicina y Salud Publica* (Septermber 5, 2019) http://medicinaysaludpublica.com/ testosterone-insufficiency-and-treatment-in-women-international-expert-consensus.

Jones, T. Hugh, et al. "The effects of testosterone on risk factors for, and the mediators of, the atherosclerotic process." *Atherosclerosis* 207, no. 2, (2009): 318–327.

Maclaren, K., et al. "The safety of post-menopausal testosterone therapy." *Women's Health* (2012): 263–275.

Shufelt, C. L., and G. D. Braunstein. "Testosterone and the breast." *Menopause International* 14, no. 3 (2008): 117–122. https://doi.org/10.1258/mi.2008.008015.

Syme, M. R., et al. "Drug transfer and metabolism by the human placenta." *Clinical Pharmacokinetics* 43 (2004): 487–514.

Wilson, C. M., and M. J. McPhaul. "A and B forms of the androgen receptor are expressed in a variety of human tissues." *Molecular and Cellular Endocrinology* 120 (1996): 51–57.

Chapter Two

Dimitrakakis, C., R. Glaser, and A. York. "Beneficial effects of testosterone therapy in women measured by the validated Menopause Rating Scale (MRS)." *Maturitas* 68, no. 4 (2011): 355–361.

Grindler, Natalia M., Jenifer E. Allsworth, George A. Macones, Kurunthachalam Kannan, Kimberly A. Roehl, and Amber R. Cooper. "Persistent Organic Pollutants and Early Menopause in U.S. Women." *PLOS One* 10, no. 1 (2015) https://doi.org/10.1371/journal.pone.0116057.

http://chemindigest.com/leopold-ruzicka-1887-1976/.

https://www.goldjournal.net/article/S0090-4295(14)01126-1/pdf.

Meeker, John D., and Kelly K. Ferguson. "Urinary Phthalate Metabolites Are Associated with Decreased Serum Testosterone in Men, Women, and Children from NHANES 2011–2012." *Journal of Clinical Endocrinology & Metabolism* (2014): 2014–2555. doi: 10.1210/jc.2014-2555.

Sarrel, P., et al. "The Mortality Toll of Estrogen Avoidance: An Analysis of Excess Deaths Among Hysterectomized Women Aged 50 to 59 Years." *American Journal of Public Health* (July 18, 2013): e1–e6.

Sherwin, Barbara B., et al. "Differential symptom response to parenteral estrogen and/or androgen administration in the surgical menopause." *American Journal of Obstetrics & Gynecology* 151, no. 2 (1965): 153–160.

Chapter Three

Bell, James R., Kimberley M. Mellor, Amanda C. Wollermann, Wendy T. K. Ip, Melissa E. Reichelt, Sarah J. Meachem, Evan R. Simpson, and Lea M. D. Delbridge. "Aromatase Deficiency Confers Paradoxical Postischemic Cardioprotection." *Endocrinology* 152, no. 12 (December 1, 2011): 4937–4947. https://doi.org/10.1210/en.2011-1212.

https://www.cdc.gov/heartdisease/women.htm.

https://health.usnews.com/health-care/patient-advice/slideshows/7-major-gaps-in-womens-health-research?slide=8.

https://www.menopause.org/for-women/menopauseflashes/bone-health-and-heart-health/keeping-your-heart-healthy-at-menopause.

LaRosa, John C. "Lipids and cardiovascular disease: Do the findings and therapy apply equally to men and women?" *Women's Health Issues* 2, no. 2: 102–113.

Matthews, K. A., S. L. Crawford, C. U. Chae, et al. "Are changes in cardiovascular disease risk factors in midlife women due to chronological aging or to the menopausal transition?" *Journal of the American College of Cardiology* 54, no. 25 (2009): 2366–2373. doi:10.1016/j.jacc.2009.10.009.

Naessen, Tord, Ulrika Sjogren, Jonas Bergquist, Marita Larsson, Lars Lind, and Mark M. Kushnir. "Endogenous Steroids Measured by High-Specificity Liquid Chromatography-Tandem Mass Spectrometry and Prevalent Cardiovascular Disease in 70-Year-Old Men and Women." *Journal of Clinical Endocrinology & Metabolism* 95, no. 4 (April 1, 2010): 1889–97. https://doi.org/10.1210/jc.2009-1722.

Pergola, C., A. Rogge, G. Dodt, H. Northoff, C. Weinigel, D. Barz, O. Radmark, L. Sautebin, and O. Werz. "Testosterone suppresses phospholipase D, causing sex differences in leukotriene biosynthesis in human monocytes." *The FASEB Journal* (2011). doi: 10.1096/fj.11-182758.

Rajendran, P., T. Rengarajan, J. Thangavel, et al. "The vascular endothelium and human diseases." *International Journal of Biological Sciences* 9, no. 10 (November 9, 2013): 1057–69. doi:10.7150/ijbs.7502.

Zieske, A. W., G. T. Malcom, and J. P. Strong. "Natural history and risk factors of atherosclerosis in children and youth: the PDAY study." *Pediatric Pathology & Molecular Medicine* 21, no. 2 (Mar–April 2002): 213–37.

Chapter Four

Alzheimer's Association, *2019 Alzheimer's Disease Facts and Figures.*

Dart, D. A., J. Waxman, E. O. Aboagye, and C. L. Bevan. "Visualising androgen receptor activity in male and female mice." *PLOS One* 8, no. 8 (August 7, 2013) https://doi.org/10.1371/journal.pone.0071694.

Endocrine Society. "Testosterone improves verbal learning and memory in postmenopausal women." *ScienceDaily* (June 17, 2013). www.sciencedaily.com/releases/2013/06/130617142043.htm.

Friedman, E. *How You and Your Doctor Can Fight Breast Cancer, Prostate Cancer, and Alzheimer's.* New York: Prometheus, 2013.

Gouras G. K., H. Xu, R. S. Gross, et al. "Testosterone reduces neuronal secretion of Alzheimer's beta-amyloid peptides." *Proceedings of the National Academy of Sciences of the United States of America* 97, no. 3 (2009): 1202–1205. doi:10.1073/pnas.97.3.1202.

Scheyer, O., A. Rahman, H. Hristov, et al. "Female Sex and Alzheimer's Risk: The Menopause Connection." *Journal of Prevention of Alzheimer's Disease* 5, no. 4 (2018): 225–230. doi:10.14283/jpad.2018.34.

University of California–San Francisco. "Testosterone Aids Older Men's Brains, UCSF Study Says." *ScienceDaily* (April 16, 2002). www.sciencedaily.com/releases/2002/04/020416073158.htm.

Chapter Five

Cooper, A., and B. B. Cooper. *A treatise on dislocations, and on fractures of the joints.* London: Churchill, 1822.

Davison, S. "Androgens in Women." *Journal of Steroid Biochemistry & Molecular Biology* 85 (2003): 363–366.

Florencio-Silva, Rinaldo, Gisela Rodrigues da Silva Sasso, Estela Sasso-Cerri, Manuel Jesus Simões, and Paulo Sérgio Cerri. "Biology of Bone Tissue: Structure, Function, and Factors That Influence

Bone Cells." *BioMed Research International* 2015, no. 421746 (2015) https://doi.org/10.1155/2015/421746.

International Osteoporosis Foundation, https://www.iofbonehealth.org.

Lovejoy, J. C., F. A. Bray, M. O. Bourgeois, R. Macchiavelli, J. C. Rood, C. Greesen, and C. Partington. "Exogenous androgens influence body composition and regional body fat distribution in obese post-menopausal women—a clinical research center study." *Journal of Clinical Endocrinology & Metabolism* 81 (1996): 2198–2203.

Manolagas, S. C., C. A. O'Brien, and M. Almeida. "The role of estrogen and androgen receptors in bone health and disease." *Nature Reviews Endocrinology* 9, no. 12 (2013): 699–712. doi:10.1038/nrendo.2013.179.

Notelovitz, Morris. "Androgen effects on bone and muscle." *Fertility and Sterility* 77 (2002): 34–41.

Office of the Surgeon General. "Bone health and osteoporosis: A report of the Surgeon General." Rockville: US Department of Health and Human Services, 2004.

Raisz L.G. "Pathogenesis of Osteoporosis." *Journal of Clinical Investigation* 115, no. 12 (2005): 3318–25.

Savvas, M., J. W. Studd, S. Norman, A. T. Leather, T. J. Garnett, and I. Fogelman. "Increase in bone mass after one year of percutaneous oestradiol and testosterone implants in post-menopausal women who have previously received long-term oral oestrogens." *BJOG: An International Journal of Obstetrics & Gynaecology* 99 (1992): 757–760. doi:10.1111/j.1471-0528.1992.tb13879.x.

Studd, J., et al. "The relationship between plasma estradiol and the increase in bone density in postmenopausal women after treatment with subcutaneous hormone implants." *American Journal of Obstetrics & Gynecology* 163, no. 5 (1990): 1474–79.

University of Gothenburg, "Keeping active in middle age may be tied to lower risk of dementia." *ScienceDaily* (February 25, 2019). www.sciencedaily.com/releases/2019/02/190225145650.htm.

Chapter Six

Aliano, Steven. "Women's Pain: Taking a Closer Look at the Disparity." *Practical Pain Management* (August 14, 2018). https://www.practi-

calpainmanagement.com/patient/resources/pain-self-management/
women-pain-taking-closer-look-disparity.

Aloisi, A. M., V. Bachiocco, A. Costantino, R. Stefani, I. Ceccarelli, A.
Bertaccini, and M. C. Meriggiola. "Cross-sex hormone administration changes pain in transsexual women and men." *Pain* 132,
supplement 1 (2007): 60–67.

Bianchi, V. E. "The Anti-Inflammatory Effects of Testosterone," *Journal
of the Endocrine Society* 3, no. 1 (October 22, 2018): 91–107.
doi:10.1210/js.2018-00186.

Coluzzi, F., D. Billeci, M. Maggi, and G. Corona. "Testosterone
deficiency in non-cancer opioid-treated patients." *Journal of
Endocrinological Investigation* 41, no. 12 (2018): 1377–1388.
doi:10.1007/s40618-018-0964-3.

Duarte, R. V., J. H. Raphael, J. L. Southall, M. H. Labib, A. J. Whallett,
and R. L. Ashford. "Hypogonadism and low bone mineral density
in patients on long-term intrathecal opioid delivery therapy." *BMJ
Open* 3, no. 6 (2013): ii. e002856.

Forman, L. J., V. Tingle, S. Estilow, and J. Cater. "The response to anal-
gesia testing is affected by gonadal steroids in the rat." *Life Science*
45, no. 5 (1989): 447–454.

Gibson, Carolyn J., PhD, MPH, Yongmei Li, PhD, Daniel Bertenthal,
MPH, Alison J. Huang, MD, MAS, and Karen H. Seal, MD,
MPH. "Menopause symptoms and chronic pain in a national
sample of midlife women veterans." *Menopause* 26, no. 7 (July
2019): 708–713. doi: 10.1097/GME.0000000000001312.

Jung-Ho, P., et al. *BMJ Open* 7, no. 11 (2017).

Koelling, Sebastian, and Nicolai Miosge. "Sex Differences of Chondro-
genic Progenitor Cells in Late Stages of Osteoarthritis." *Arthritis &
Rheumatism* 62, no. 4 (January 13, 2010): 1077-87.

Mensah-Nyagan, A. G., L. Meyer, V. Schaeffer, C. Kibaly, and C.
Patte-Mensah. "Evidence for a key role of steroids in the modula-
tion of pain." *Psychoneuroendocrinology* 34, supplement 1 (2009):
S169–S177.

Stoffel, E. C., C. M. Ulibarri, J. E. Folk, K. C. Rice, and R. M. Craft.
"Gonadal hormone modulation of mu, kappa, and delta opioid

antinociception in male and female rats." *Journal of Pain* 6, no. 4 (2005): 261–274.

Tennant, Forest, MD, PhD. "Hormone Therapies: Newest Advance in Pain Care." *Practical Pain Management* 11, no. 4 (2011): 98-105.

VanHouten, J. P., R. A. Rudd, M. F. Ballesteros, and K. A. Mack. "Drug Overdose Deaths Among Women Aged 30–64 Years—United States, 1999–2017." *Morbidity and Mortality Weekly Report* 68 (2019): 1–5. http://dx.doi.org/10.15585/mmwr.mm6801a1external icon.

White, H., et al. "Treatment of Pain in Fibromyalgia Patients With Testosterone Gel: Pharmacokinetics and Clinical Response." *International Immunopharmacology* 27, no. 2 (2015): 249–56.

Zhang, Y., and J. M. Jordan. "Epidemiology of osteoarthritis" (published correction appears in *Clinics in Geriatric Medicine.* 29, no. 2 (May 2013): ix). *Clinics in Geriatric Medicine* 26, no. 3 (2010): 355–369. doi:10.1016/j.cger.2010.03.001.

Chapter Seven

Adair, F., and J. Herrmann. "The use of testosterone propionate in the treatment of advanced carcinoma of the breast." *Annals of Surgery* 123 (1946): 1023–35.

Agoff, S., P. Swanson, H. Linden, S. Hawes, and T. Lawton. "Androgen receptor expression in estrogen receptor-negative breast cancer." *American Journal of Clinical Pathology* 120 (2003): 725–31.

Agrawal, A., M. Jelen, Z. Grzelenek, et al. "Androgen Receptor as a prognostic and predictive factor in breast cancer." *Folia Histochemica et Cytobiologica* 46 (2008): 269–276.

American College of Obstetricians and Gynecologists. "ACOG Practice Bulletin: Breast cancer risk assessment and screening in average risk women." (2017). Retrieved from https://www.acog.org/Clinical-Guidance-and-Publications/Practice-Bulletins/Committee-on-Practice-Bulletins-Gynecology/Breast-Cancer-Risk-Assessment-and-Screening-in-Average-Risk-Women.

Ando, S., F. De Amicis, V. Rago, A. Carpino, M. Maggiolini, M. Panno, and M. Lanzino. "Breast cancer from estrogen to androgen receptor." *Molecular and Cellular Endocrinology* 19 (2002): 121–128.

Breastcancer.org. "Types of breast cancer." (2018). Retrieved from https://www.breastcancer.org/symptoms/types.

Cheang, M., S. Chia, D. Voduc, D. Gao, S. Leung, J. Snider, et al. "Ki67 index, HER2 status, and prognosis in patients with luminal B breast cancer." *Journal of the National Cancer Institute* 101 (2009): 736–750.

Choi, J., S. Kang, S. Lee, and Y. Bae. "Androgen receptor expression predicts decrease survival in early stage TNBC." *Annals of Surgical Oncology* 22, no. 1 (2015): 82–89.

Collins, L., K. Cole, J. Marotti, R. Hu, S. Schnitt, and R. Tamimi. "Androgen receptor in breast cancer in relation to the molecular phenotype." *Modern Pathology* 24 (2011): 924–931.

Dimitrakakis, C., J. Zhou, and J. Wang. "A physiologic role for testosterone limiting estrogenic stimulation of the breast." *Menopause* 10 (2003): 292–298.

Dimitrakakis, C., R. Jones, A. Liu, and C. Bondy. "Breast cancer incidence in postmenopausal women using testosterone in addition to usual hormone therapy." *Menopause* 11 (2004): 531–535.

Dimitrakakis, C., D. Zava, S. Marinopoulous, A. Tsigginou, A. Antsaklis, and R. Glaser. "Low salivary testosterone levels in patients with breast cancer." *BMC Cancer* 10 (2010): 547.

Friedman E. *The New Testosterone Treatment.* Buffalo: Prometheus Books, 2013.

Glaser, R. "Reduced breast cancer incidence in women treated with subcutaneous testosterone." *Maturitas* 76 (2013): 342–349.

Glaser, R. L., A. E. York, and C. Dimitrakakis. "Abstract P6-13-02: Reduced incidence of breast cancer with testosterone implant therapy: A 10-year cohort study." *Cancer Research* 79, supplement 4 (February 15, 2019): P6-13-02. doi:10.1158/1538-7445. SABCS18-P6-13-02.

Glaser, Rebecca, and Constantine Dimitrakakis. "Rapid response of breast cancer to neoadjuvant intramammary testosterone-anastrozole therapy: neoadjuvant hormone therapy in breast cancer." *Menopause* (June 1, 2014).

Grann, V., K. Panageas, W. Whang, et al. "Decision analysis of prophylactic mastectomy and oophorectomy in BRCA1-positive or BRCA2-positive patients." *Journal of Clinical Oncology* 16, no. 3 (1998): 979–985.

Henderson, B. "Hormonal Carcinogenesis," *Carcinogenesis* 21, no. 3 (2000): 427–433.

Herrmann, J., and F. Adair. "The effects of testosterone propionate on carcinoma of the female breast with soft tissue metastasis." *Journal of Clinical Endocrinology & Metabolism* 6 (1946): 769–775.

Hilborn, E. "Androgen receptor expression predicts beneficial tamoxifen response." *British Journal of Cancer* 114 (2016): 248–255.

Hofling, M., A. Hirschberg, L. Skoog, et al. "Testosterone inhibits estrogen/progestogen-induced breast cell proliferation in postmenopausal women." *Menopause* 14 (2007): 183.

Howlader, N., A. Noone, M. Krapcho, D. Miller, K. Bishop, C. Kosary, et al. "SEER Cancer Statistics Review, 1975–2014." https://seer.cancer.gov/csr/1975_2014, based on November 2016 SEER data submission.

Kuchenbaecker, K., J. Hopper, D. Barnes, et al. "Risks of breast, ovarian, and contralateral breast cancer for BRCA1 and BRCA2 mutation carriers." *Journal of the American Medical Association* 317, no. 23 (2017): 2402–2416.

Lehmann, B., J. Bauer, J. Schafer, C. Pendleton, L. Tang, K. Johnson, et al. "PIK3CA mutations in androgen receptor positive triple negative breast cancer confers sensitivity to the combination of PI3K and androgen receptor inhibitors." *Breast Cancer Research* (2014).

Leylan-Jones, B. "Human Epidermal growth factor receptor 2 positive breast cancers and CNS metastasis." *Journal of Clinical Oncology* 27 (2009): 5278–86.

Longo, D., A. Fauci, D. Kasper, S. Hauser, and J. Jameson. *Harrison's Principles of Internal Medicine*, 18th edition. New York: McGraw Hill, 2011.

McNamara, K. M., T. Yoda, Y. Miki, N. Chanplakorn, S. Wongwaisayawan, P. Incharoen, et al. "Androgen pathway in triple negative invasive ductal tumors." *Cancer Sciience* 104 (2013): 639–646.

Metcalfe, K., S. Gershman, P. Ghadirian, H. Lynch, C. Snyder, N. Tung, et al. "Contralateral mastectomy and survival after breast cancer in carriers of BRCA1 and BRCA2 mutations: retrospective analysis." *British Medical Journal* (2014): 348.

Narayanan, R., and T. Dalton. "Androgen Receptor: A complex therapeutic target for breast cancer." *Cancers* 8 (2016): 108–125.

Nathanson, K. "Breast Cancer Genetics." *Natural Medicine* 7 (2015): 552–556.

National Cancer Institute. "Breast cancer treatment." (2018). Retrieved from https://www.cancer.gov/types/breast/hp/breast-treatment-pdq.

Noh, S., J. Kim, and J. Koo. "Metabolic differences in estrogen receptor negative breast cancer is based on androgen receptor status." *Tumor Biol* 35 (2014): 8179–92.

Onitilo, A., J. Engel, R. Greenlee, and B. Mukesh. "Breast cancer subtypes based on ER/PR and HER2 expression." *Clinical Medical Research* 7 (2009): 4–13.

Perou, C., T. Sorlie, M. Eisen, M. van de Rijn, S. Jeffrey, C. Rees, et. al. "Molecular portraits of human breast tumors." *Nature* 407 (2000): 748–752.

Peters, A., G. Buchanan, C. Ricciardelli, T. Bianco-Miotto, M. Centenera, J. Harris, et al. "Androgen receptor inhibits estrogen receptor-alpha activity and is prognostic in breast cancer." *Cancer Research* 69 (2009): 6131–40.

Qu, Q., Y. Mao, X. Fei, and K. Shen. "The impact of the androgen receptor expression on breast cancer survival." *PLOS One* 8 (2013): 1-8.

Santen, R., W. Uyue, and D. Heitan. "Modeling of the growth kinetics of occult breast tumors." *Cancer Epidemiology, Biomarkers and Prevention* 21, no. 7 (2012): 1038–48.

Siegel, R., K. Miller, and A. Jemal. "Cancer Statistics, 2018." *CA: A Cancer Journal for Clinicians* 68, no. 1 (2018): 7–30.

"The Manchester guidelines for contralateral risk-reducing mastectomy." Available from: https://www.researchgate.net/publication/280911 207_The_Manchester_guidelines_for_contralateral_risk-reducing_mastectomy (accessed December 10, 2018), PDF.

U.S. Preventive Services Task Force (USPSTF), "Breast cancer risk assessment, genetic counseling, & genetic testing." (2013).

Retrieved from https://www.uspreventiveservicestaskforce.org/Page/ Document/UpdateSummaryFinal/brca-related-cancer-risk-assess- ment-genetic-counseling-and-genetic-testing.

Vera-Badillo, F. E., A. Templeton, P. deGouveia, I. Diaz-Padilla, P. Bedard, M. Al-Mubarak, et al. "Androgen receptor expression and outcomes in early breast cancer." *Journal of the National Cancer Institute* (2014).

Walsh-Childers, K., H. Edwards, and S. Grobmyer. "Covering women's greatest health fear: Breast cancer information in consumer maga- zines." *Health Communication* 26, no. 3 (2011): 1–12, 209—220.

Chapter Eight

Abraham, G.E. "Facts about iodine and autoimmune thyroiditis." *The Original Internist* 15, no. 2 (2008): 75–76.

Barnes, B., and L. Galton. *Hypothyroidism: The unsuspected illness.* Canada: Fitzhenry & Whiteside Limited, 1976.

Bauer, D. C. "Low thyrotropin levels are not associated with bone loss in older women: a prospective study." *Journal of Clinical Endocrinology & Metabolism* 82, no. 9 (1997): 2931–6.

Biondi, B. "The normal TSH reference range: What has changed in the last decade?" *Journal of Clinical Endocrinology & Metabolism* 98, no. 9 (2013): 3584–3587.

Cerillo, A., S. Bevilacqua, S. Storti, M. Mariani, E. Kallushi, A. Ripoli, et al. "Free triiodothyronine: a novel predictor of postoperative atrial fibrillation." *European Journal of Cardiothoracic Surgery* 24, no. 4 (2003): 487–492.

Chardes, T., N. Chapal, D. Bresson, C. Bes, V. Giudicelli, M. P. Lefranc, et al. "The human anti-thyroidperoxidase autoantibody repertoire in Graves' and Hashimoto's autoimmune thyroid diseases." *Immu- nogenetics* 54 (2002): 141–57.

Christ-Crain, M., C. Meier, M. Guglielmetti, P. R. Huber, W. Riesen, J. Staubb, and B. Muller. "Elevated C-reactive protein and homo- cysteine values: cardiovascular risk factors in hypothyroidism? A cross-sectional and a double-blind, placebo-controlled trial." *Athero- sclerosis* 166, no. 2 (2003): 379–386.

Danzi, S., and I. Klein. "Potential uses of T3 in the treatment of human disease." *Clinical Cornerstone* 7, supplement 2 (2005): S9–15.

Dunn, Donna, PhD, CNM, FNP-BC (assistant professor), and Carla Turner, DNP, ACNP-BC (instructor). "Hypothyroidism in Women." Nursing For Women's Health, vol. 20 (2016): 93-96.

El Hadidy, E. M., et al. "Impact of severity, duration and etiology of hyperthyroidism on bone turnover markers and bone mineral density in men." *BMC Endocrine Disorders* 11 (2011): 2–7.

Elhomsy, G., and E. Staros, eds. "Antithyroid Antibody." *Laboratory Medicine* (2014).

Escobar-Morreale, H. F., et al. "Replacement therapy for hypothyroidism with thyroxine alone does not ensure euthyroidism in all tissues, as studied in thyroidectomized rats." *Journal of Clinical Investigation* 96, no. 6 (1995): 2828–38.

Escobar-Morreale, H. F., F. E. del Rey, M. J. Obregon, and G. M. de Escobar. "Only the combined treatment with thyroxine and triiodothyronine ensures euthyroidism in all tissues of the thyroidectomized rat." *Endocrinology* 137, no. 6 (1996): 2490–2502.

Fraser, W. D., D. Biggart, St. J. O'Reilly, H. W. Gray, J. H. McKillop, and J. A. Thompson. "Are biochemical tests of thyroid function of any value in monitoring patients receiving thyroxine therapy?" *British Medical Journal* 293 (1986): 1373.

Garin, M. C. "Subclinical thyroid dysfunction and hip fracture and bone mineral density in older adults: The cardiovascular health study." *Journal of Clinical Endocrinology & Metabolism* 99, no. 8 (2014): 2657–64.

Gartner, R. "Selenium supplementation in patients with autoimmune thyroiditis decreases thyroid peroxidase antibodies concentrations." *Journal of Clinical Endocrinology & Metabolism* 87, no. 4 (2002): 1687–91.

Gorres, G., et al. "Bone mineral density in patients receiving suppressive doses of thyroxine for differentiated thyroid carcinoma." *European Journal of Nuclear Medicine* 23, no. 6 (1996): 690–692.

Heijckmann, A. C. "Hip bone mineral density, bone turnover and risk of fracture in patients on long-term suppressive L-thyroxine therapy for differentiated thyroid carcinoma." *European Journal of Endocrinology* 153, no. 1 (2005): 23–29.

Hennemann, R. D., E. Friesema, et al. "Plasma membrane transport of thyroid hormones and its role in thyroid hormone metabolism and bioavailability." *Endocrine Reviews* 22, no. 4 (2001): 451–476.

Hoang, T. D., C. H. Olsen, V. Q. Mai, P. W. Clyde, and M. K. Shakir. "Desiccated thyroid extract compared with levothyroxine in the treatment of hypothyroidism: A randomized, double-blind, crossover study." *Journal of Clinical Endocrinology & Metabolism* 98, no. 5 (2013): 1982–90.

Jameson, J., A. Fauci, D. Kasper, S. Hauser, D. Longo, and J. Loscalzo, eds. *Harrison's Principles of Internal Medicine*, 20th edition. New York: McGraw Hill, 2018.

Kharrazian, D. *Why do I still have thyroid symptoms when my lab tests are normal: A revolutionary breakthrough in understanding Hashimoto's disease and hypothyroidism.* New York: Morgan James Publishing, 2010.

Krotkiewski, M. "Thyroid hormones and treatment of obesity." *International Journal of Obesity* 24 (2000): S116–S119.

Larsen, P. R. "Thyroid-pituitary interaction: feedback regulation of thyrotropin secretion by thyroid hormones." *New England Journal of Medicine* 306, no. 1 (1982): 23–32.

Lim, V. S., C. Passo, Y. Murata, E. Ferrari, et al. "Reduced triiodothyronine content in liver but not pituitary of the uremic rat model: demonstration of changes compatible with thyroid hormone deficiency in liver only." *Endocrinology* 114, no. 1 (1984): 280–286.

Lu, R., K. Burman, and J. Jonklaas. "Transient Graves' hyperthyroidism during pregnancy in a patient with Hashimoto's hypothyroidism." *Thyroid* 15, no. 7 (2005): 725–9.

Luidens, M., S. Mousa, F. Davis, H. Lin, and P. Davis. "Thyroid hormone and angiogenesis." *Vascular Pharmacology* 52, no. 3-4 (2010): 142–145.

Maia, A. L., et al. "Pituitary cells respond to thyroid hormone by discrete, gene-specific pathways." *Endocrinology* 136 (1995): 1488–94.

Mazziotti, G., L. D. Premawardhana, A. Parkes, H. Adams, P. Smyth, D. Smith, W. Kaluarachi, et al. "Evolution of thyroid autoimmunity during iodine prophylaxis—the Sri Lankan experience." *European Journal of Endocrinology* 149 (2003): 103–110.

Nedrebo, B., U. Ericsson, H. Nygard, et al. "Plasma total homocysteine levels in hyperthyroid and hypothyroid patients." *Metabolism* 47, no. 1 (1998): 89–93.

Ohye, H., E. Nishihara, I. Sasaki, et al. "Four cases of Graves' disease which developed after painful Hashimoto's thyroiditis." *Internal Medicine* 45 (2006): 385–389.

Ortiga-Carvalho, T. M., et al. "Thyroid hormone receptors and resistance to thyroid hormone disorders." *National Review of Endocrinology* 10, no. 10 (2014): 582–591.

Pavlou, H., P. Kliridis, A. Panagiotopoulos, C. Goritsas, and P. Vassilakos. "Euthyroid sick syndrome in acute ischemic syndromes." *Angiology* 53, no. 6 (2002): 699–707.

Pepper, G. M., and P. Y. Casanova-Romero. "Conversion to Armour Thyroid from Levothyroxine improved patient satisfaction in the treatment of hypothyroidism." *Journal of Endocrinology, Diabetes, and Obesity* 2, no. 3 (2014): 1055.

Persani, L. "Central Hypothyroidism: Pathogenic, diagnostic, and therapeutic challenges." *Journal of Clinical Endocrinology & Metabolism* 9, no. 7 (2012): 3068–78.

Peterson, S. J., A. Cappola, R. Castro, C. Dayan, A. Farwell, J. Hennessey, et al. "An Online Survey of Hypothyroid Patients Demonstrates Prominent Dissatisfaction." *Thyroid* (2018). (e-pub ahead of print) doi: 10.1089/thy.2017.0681.

Quan, M. L. "Bone mineral density in well-differentiated thyroid cancer patients treated with suppressive thyroxine: A systematic overview of the literature." *Journal of Surgical Oncology* 79, no. 1 (2002): 62–70.

Reverter, J. L. "Lack of deleterious effect on bone mineral density of long-term thyroxine suppressive therapy for differentiated thyroid carcinoma." *Endocrine-Related Cancer* 12, no. 4 (2005): 973–981.

Rosen, H. N. "Randomized trial of pamidronate in patients with thyroid cancer: bone density is not reduced by suppressive doses of thyroxine but is increased by cyclic intravenous pamidronate." *Journal of Clinical Endocrinology and Metabolism* 83, no. 7 (1998): 2324–30

Saravanan, P., and C. M. Dayan. "Thyroid autoantibodies." *Endocrinology and Metabolism Clinics of North America* 30 (2001): 315–337.

Sheppard, M. C."Levothyroxine treatment and occurrence of fracture of the hip." *Archives of Internal Medicine* 162, no. 3 (2002): 338–343.

Shimoyama, *Cardiology* (1993).

Starr, M., *Hypothyroidism type 2: The epidemic.* Irvine: New Voice Publication, 2011.

Strich, D., G. Karavani, S. Edri, and D. Gillis. "TSH enhancement of FT4 to FT3 conversion is age dependent." *European Journal of Endocrinology* 175 (2016): 49–54.

Van Den Eeden, S. K. "Thyroid hormone use and the risk of hip fracture in women >/=65 years: A case-control study." *Journal of Women's Health (Larchmt)* 12, no. 1 (2003): 27–31.

Wentz, I., and M. Nowosadzka. *Hashimoto's thyroiditis: Lifestyle interventions for finding and treating the root cause.* White River Junction: Wentz, LLC, 2013.

Yingheng, L., B. Sherer, A. Redetzke, and M. Gerdes. "Regulation of arteriolar density in adult myocardium during low thyroid conditions." *Vascular Pharmacology* 52, no. 3–4 (2010): 146–150.

Chapter Nine

Ambler, D. R., E. J. Bieber, and M. P. Diamond. "Sexual function in elderly women: a review of current literature." *Reviews in Obstetrics Gynecology* 5, no. 1 (2012): 16–27.

Goldstein, Irwin, et al. "Hypoactive Sexual Desire Disorder." *Mayo Clinic Proceedings* 92, no. 1 (2017): 114–128.

https://www.mayoclinic.org/diseases-conditions/erectile-dysfunction/symptoms-causes/syc-20355776.

Islam, R. M., R. J. Bell, S. Green, and S. R. Davis. "Effects of testosterone therapy for women: a systematic review and meta-analysis protocol." *Systematic Reviews* 8, no. 1 (January 11, 2019). doi:10.1186/s13643-019-0941-8.

Kim, H. K., S. Y. Kang, Y. J. Chung, J. H. Kim, and M. R. Kim. "The Recent Review of the Genitourinary Syndrome of Menopause." *Journal of Menopausal Medicine* 21, no. 2 (2015): 65–71. doi:10.6118/jmm.2015.21.2.65.

Levkovich, I., A. Gewirtz-Meydan, K. Karkabi, and L. Ayalon. "When sex meets age: Family physicians' perspectives about sexual dysfunction among older men and women: A qualitative study from Israel." *European Journal of General Practice* 25, no. 2 (2019): 85–90. doi:10.1080/13814788.2019.1580263.

Nappi, Rossella E., et al. "The CLOSER (CLarifying Vaginal Atrophy's Impact On SEx and Relationships) Survey: Implications of Vaginal Discomfort in Postmenopausal Women and in Male Partners." *The Journal of Sexual Medicine* 10, no. 9: 2232–41.

———. "Women's perception of sexuality around the menopause: Outcomes of a European telephone survey." *European Journal of Obstetrics and Gynecology and Reproductive Biology* 137, no. 1 ( ): 10–16.

Scavello, I., E. Maseroli, V. Di Stasi, and L. Vignozzi. "Sexual Health in Menopause." *Medicina (Kaunas)* 55, no. 9 (September 2, 2019): 559. doi:10.3390/medicina55090559.

Simon, James, Irwin Goldstein, Noel Kim, et al. "The role of androgens in the treatment of genitourinary syndrome of menopause (GSM): International Society for the Study of Women's Sexual Health (ISSWSH) expert consensus panel review." *Menopause* (July 1, 2018). http://www.sciencedirect.com/science/article/pii/S2050052118300465.

Traish, Abdulmaged M., Linda Vignozzi, James A. Simon, Irwin Goldstein, and Noel N. Kim. "Role of Androgens in Female Genitourinary Tissue Structure and Function: Implications in the Genitourinary Syndrome of Menopause." *Sexual Medicine Reviews* 6, no. 4 (2018): 558. https://doi.org/10.1016/j.sxmr.2018.03.005.

Chapter Ten

Glaser, Rebecca, et al. "Testosterone therapy in women: Myths and misconceptions." *Maturitas* 74, no. 3: 230–234.

Chapter Eleven

Aspinall, Mara G., and Richard G. Hamermesh. "Realizing the Promise of Personalized Medicine." *Harvard Business Review* (October 2007).

Carruthers, M., T.R. Trinick, and M.J. Wheeler. "The validity of androgen assays." *Aging Male* 10 (2007):165-72.

Elliott, Ivo, Mayfong Mayxay, Sengchanh Yeuichaixong, Sue J. Lee, and Paul N. Newton. "The practice and clinical implications of tablet splitting in international health." *Tropical Medicine & International Health* 19, no. 7 (July 2014): 754–760. (published online April 7, 2014) doi: 10.1111/tmi.12309. PMCID: PMC4285309.

Princeton Consensus Group. "Fertility and Sterility." (2002).

Chapter Twelve

Davis, Susan R. "Is testosterone important for women as they age?" *Maturitas* 100 (2017): 95.

Davison, S. L., R. Bell, S. Donath, J. G. Montalto, and S. R. Davis. "Androgen levels in adult females: changes with age, menopause, and oophorectomy." *Journal of Clinical Endocrinology & Metabolism* 90 (2005): 3847–3850.

North American Menopause Society. "Hormone Therapy Position Statement of the North American Menopause Society." *The Journal of the North American Menopause Society* 24, no. 7 (2017): 728–753.

Slomski A. "Which Postmenopausal Women Should Use Testosterone for Low Sexual Desire?" *Journal of the American Medical Association.* (published online January 22, 2020) doi:10.1001/jama.2019.22070.

Chapter Thirteen

Collins, P. "Effects of testosterone on Coronary Vasomotor Regulation." *Circulation* 100 (1999): 1690–1696.

Feldman, Henry A., Christopher Longcope, Carol A. Derby, Catherine B. Johannes, Andre B. Araujo, Andrea D. Coviello, William J. Bremner, and John B. McKinlay. "Age Trends in the Level of Serum Testosterone and Other Hormones in Middle-Aged Men: Longitudinal Results from the Massachusetts Male Aging Study." *Journal of Clinical Endocrinology & Metabolism* 87, no. 2 (February 1, 2002): 589–598.

Finkle, W. D., S. Greenland, G. K. Ridgeway, et al. "Increased risk of non-fatal myocardial infarction following testosterone therapy prescription in men." *PLOS One* 9, no. 1 (January 29, 2014) doi:10.1371/journal.pone.0085805.

Khaw, Kay-Tee, Mitch Dowsett, Elizabeth Folkerd, Sheila Bingam, Nicholas Wareham, Robert Luben, Ailsa Welch, and Nicholas Day. "Endogenous Testosterone and Mortality Due to All Causes, Cardiovascular Disease, and Cancer in Men, European Prospective Investigation into Cancer in Norfolk (EPIC-Norfolk) Prospective Population Study." *Circulation* 116 (November 26, 2007): 2694–2701. https://doi.org/10.1161/CIRCULATIONAHA.107.719005.

Mearini, L., A. Zucchi, et al. "Prevalence of low testosterone (total testosterone less than 300 ng/dl) is as high as 38.7% in males over 45 in out-patient primary care populations." *World Journal of Urology* 31, no. 2 (November 9, 2011): 247–252.

Morgentaler, Abraham, et al. "Fundamental Concepts Regarding Testosterone Deficiency and Treatment." *Mayo Clinic Proceedings* 91, no. 7 (2016): 881–896.

Mulligan, T., M. F. Frick, Q. C. Zuraw, A. Stemhagen, and C. McWhirter. "Prevalence of hypogonadism in males aged at least 45 years: the HIM study." *International Journal of Clinical Practice* 60, no. 7 (2006): 762–769. doi:10.1111/j.1742-1241.2006.00992.x.

Pastuszak, A. W. "Testosterone replacement therapy in patients with prostate cancer after radical prostatectomy." *Journal of Urology* 190 (2013): 639–644.

Sharma, R., O. A. Oni, K. Gupta, et al. "Normalization of Testosterone Levels after Testosterone Replacement Therapy Is Associated With Decreased Incidence of Atrial Fibrillation." *Journal of the American Heart Association* 6, no. 5 (May 9, 2017) doi:10.1161/JAHA.116.004880.

Sharma, Rishi, Olurinde A. Oni, Kamal Gupta, Guoqing Chen, Mukut Sharma, Buddhadeb Dawn, Ram Sharma, Deepak Parashara, Virginia J. Savin, John A. Ambrose, and Rajat S. Barua. "Normalization of testosterone level is associated with reduced incidence of myocardial infarction and mortality in men." *European Heart Journal* 36, no. 40 (October 21, 2015): 2706–15.

Shores, M. M., A. M. Matsumoto, K. L. Sloan, and D. R. Kivlahan. "Low Serum Testosterone and Mortality in Male Veterans." *Archives of Internal Medicine* 166, no. 15 (2006): 1660–65. doi:10.1001/archinte.166.15.1660.

Tenover, J. S. "Effects of testosterone supplementation in the aging male." *Journal of Clinical Endocrinology & Metabolism* 75, no. 4 (October 1, 1992): 1092–98.

Vigen, R., C. I. O'Donnell, A. E. Barón, et al. "Association of Testosterone Therapy with Mortality, Myocardial Infarction, and Stroke in Men with Low Testosterone Levels." *Journal of the American Medical Association* 310, no. 17 (2013): 1829–36. doi:10.1001/jama.2013.280386.

Zmuda, J. *American Journal of Cardiology* 77 (1996): 1244–47.

———. *Atherosclerosis* 130 (1997): 199–202.